ANTI-INFLAMMATORY DIET AND NATURAL REMEDIES

Step by Step Guide to Reduce Inflammation, Prevent and Reverse Disease, Give Pain Relief, Improve Health and Quality of Life, Using Natural Remedies, Mindset and Relaxation Methods, Specific Food, Herbs and Spices to Easily Implement in Your Diet

By Sina Joie

Table of Contents

UNDERSTANDING INFLAMMATION

The primary thing you have to think about inflammation is that it's not all bad. Truth be told, inflammation assumes a significant job in keeping you solid. Inflammation is simply the body's method for shielding from harmful bacteria, viruses, and injury. Now and again, however, that system causes the body to turn on itself, assaulting solid cells and organs. In this section, we investigate the different kinds of inflammation and distinguish how things can turn out badly.

Understanding how the immune system reacts

The immune system is a convoluted relationship of organs, tissues, and cells that work together to ensure the body is protected. Inflammation is part of your body's response when it believes it's at risk for infection or further injury.

There are three kinds of immunity:

- Passive: Passive immunity is a brief immunity that originates from another body, for example, from the mother through the placenta or bosom milk. Inactive immunity regularly vanishes 6 months to a year after birth.

- Innate: Innate immunity is the immunity you were brought into the world. Innate immunity incorporates boundaries that prevent invaders from entering your body, just as fiery responses — hacking; creating tears, sweat, bodily fluid, and extra stomach acid, swelling, etc.

- Acquired: Acquired immunity creates within sight of certain enemies of gens. It creates as your body fabricates guards against explicit invaders, for example, viruses that cause chickenpox and the regular virus.

In this section, we spread innate and gained immunity, the two immune systems that stick around through adulthood. We talk about inflammation as part of the innate immune system, and we spread the invader-explicit resistances of the procured immune system.

Innate immunity: Providing general security with inflammation

Inflammation is part of your body's innate response to invaders. The incendiary response assumes control over when harmful bacteria, viruses, poisons, or different components advance into your tissues and cause damage. Those dam-matured cells discharge chemicals called prostaglandins and histamines, which cause veins to release liquid into the tissues and make swelling.

The subsequent inflammation — described by redness, swelling, warmth, and pain — fills in as a physical obstruction against the spread of infection (on account of disease) or against further injury (which would postpone the mending procedure). Chemical elements discharged during inflammation avoid or sharpen pain signals, making a progressively appropriate condition for mending.

Then, the immune system, detecting peril, sends backup. Different parts of the immune system react by coordinating traffic, detaching and executing the invaders, and crushing and getting out contaminated cells. The cells speak with one another through an assortment of chemical signals, including cytokines, C-receptive protein, intense stage proteins, prostaglandins, and then some. Understanding this response is useful for specialists because incendiary markers demonstrate where the issue is and how serious it might be. Analysts look at the procedure to figure out what triggers inflammation and discover approaches to control it — for example, through eating regimens — when things turn out badly.

Acquired immunity: Attacking specific invaders from past experiences

The procured, or versatile, immune system is the one you create dependent on what you do, where you go, and what you're presented to. The more bugs and viruses you interact with, the more unpredictable your procured immune system becomes.

Through a procedure called immune response, the immune system calls upon its network — cells, tissues, and organs — to battle ailment and infection. Leukocytes, or white blood cells, search out and pulverize irresistible creatures and substances. There are two kinds of leukocytes:

- Phagocytes, which are the hungry leukocytes that eat the invaders;

- Lymphocytes, which help the body distinguish and perceive attackers, so it realizes what to look for some other time.

This is what occurs: When your body recognizes antigens (the outside sub-positions), a gathering of cells get together and structure a sort of cell armed force to attack the invader. A portion of these cells produce antibodies that can lock onto the particular antigens. The antibodies fill in as labels, recognizing the invader as a foe and focusing on it for obliteration.

A portion of the antibodies keeps on living in your body so they can promptly attack if a similar antigen is recognized. Whenever the antibodies experience that antigen, they lock on and start a provocative response.

Seeing where inflammation turns out badly

At the point when inflammation works right, it attacks the irritant — the virus, harmful bacteria, or damaged cells. At times, be that as it may, the body kicks into over-drive and dispatches a hostile on ordinary, solid tissue. For instance, in the event that you have the autoimmune issue rheumatoid joint pain, you see some redness and some swelling in the joints, with joint pain and firmness. This response is an indication that your body is attempting to attack your joint tissue, which your body erroneously sees as threatening.

State your home is being surpassed by mosquitoes. You get some mosquito shower, light a citronella flame, and keep a rolled-up paper at hand. You're taking care of the irritant and the irritant as it were. Presently state, you've gone a tad over the edge. Rather than a rolled-up paper, you take a slugging stick and attempt to execute that mosquito on the wall. The issue is that the mosquito wasn't a mosquito by any means; it was only a shadow, and now you have an opening in the wall.

Similarly, the immune system can blow up to apparent dangers and damage the body.

The way your body reacts to inflammation partially relies upon your hereditary qualities and natural variables. Most by and large solid individuals respond to a cut or wound similarly, yet how the immune system reacts to a virus, a bacterium, or various nourishments can contrast from person to person. The distinctions in the way your immune system reacts rely upon the accompanying:

- Genes;

- Your overall health;

- The health of major immune organs, such as the gastrointestinal tract;

- Dietary health is affected, including nutrients and toxins in foods;

- Environmental toxins, such as pesticides;

- Deregulation of blood sugar and insulin;

- Stress factors (stress weakens the immune system).

A significant primary factor in the various ways people are influenced by inflammation is an imbalance in their procured immune systems. In a sound immune system, the helper T cells (those that are part of the immune response and attack) are in balance — one cell to attack blood-borne parasites, the other to attack invaders, for example, bacteria. As the immune system becomes overstimulated, the helper cells end up in a self-sustaining imbalance, causing the helper cells to attack the body. For whatever length of time that anything that is causing the inflammation is yet present, the imbalance remains.

Inflammation can likewise go on excessively long. The innate and the obtained immune systems speak with one another through sensors and signals, which advise the body when to discharge certain chemicals and proteins to actuate the inflammation protect. The signals should advise the inflammation when to stop also. That doesn't always occur. A few people have raised degrees of C-reactive protein, a provocative marker that leaves the body in protective mode, always prepared to attack. At the point when that occurs, your body starts a relentless descending winding prompting disease.

Making inflammation isn't something your body manages without exertion — it takes vitality, which causes fatigue and makes free radicals, atoms that cause cell damage. Because of the considerable number of things you're presented to, cells identified with the fiery response need to turn out to be entirely reliable, which implies that when they attack, they do as such with force. That force can cause damage the longer those cells are dynamic.

Understanding the distinction between acute and chronic inflammation

Inflammation might be acute or chronic. The most significant difference between the two is time:

- Acute: Acute inflammation happens very quickly after tissue damage and goes on for a brief timeframe, from a couple of moments to a few days. It's what causes wounding and swelling when you fall or sprain something.

- Chronic: Although generally not as painful as acute inflammation, chronic inflammation keeps going longer, sometimes for a while. Chronic inflammation can be caused by physical factors (viruses, bacteria, blood sugar imbalances, extraordinary warmth, or cold) or enthusiastic factors (chronic day by day stress). After some time, chronic inflammation can add to chronic disease by losing the body's immune system and making much more inflammation all the while.

A few analysts depict inflammation as high-grade or low-grade, contingent upon the seriousness of inflammation and the degrees of fiery markers, for example, C-reactive protein (CRP). Low-grade inflammation, particularly chronic low-grade inflammation, will, in general, be the more dangerous structure. Low-grade inflammation frequently prompts chronic disease, for example, atherosclerosis (solidified veins), diabetes, malignant growth, joint inflammation, different sclerosis, fractious inside disorder, hypertension, and lupus. A significant number of the factors prompting low-grade inflammation are way of life related: smoking, stress, heftiness, dormancy, and diet.

Low-grade inflammation often goes undetected, but here are common symptoms:

- Body aches and pains;

- Fever;

- Congestion;

- Frequent infections;

- Stiffness;

- Dry eyes;

- Diarrhea or irritable bowel syndrome symptoms;

- Indigestion;

- Shortness of breath;

- Fatigue.

Gut reactions: Linking food, digestion, and the immune system

For you to remain healthy, your immune system must remain healthy and in balance. Getting the right kinds and measures of proteins, fats, nutrients, and different supplements are key in getting and staying healthy. Eating right gives your body the structure blocks it needs to assemble cells and create chemicals, and the digestive system assumes a key job in the immune system.

Separating food and Dealing with the pieces

Digestion includes mechanical activities — the biting and pounding of the food — just as chemical procedures, in which compounds separate the food into minor molecules. Your body puts these molecules through a determination procedure, keeping the valuable molecules as raw materials for building cells, hormones, etc., sifting through what it can't utilize and killing and evacuating harmful substances.

Eating the right kinds of foods in the correct amounts guarantees that your body has the raw materials it needs. For instance, eating the right types of fats can fortify your immune system and assist you with fending off inflammation. Eicosanoids, which are chemicals associated with inflammation, are produced using fundamental fatty acids. Eating the right types of these fats, similar to omega-3 fatty acids, will allow your body to create mitigating eicosanoids, something that doesn't occur when you eat such a large number of omega-6 fatty acids.

Perceiving the digestive tract as part of the immune system

A significant overlooked part of the immune system is the digestive tract. Actually, 80 percent of your immune system is found there. The digestive tract contains the gut-related lymphoid tissue (GALT), a sort of tissue that screens and secures the body against pathogens (germs). There is a high centralization of GALT in the small intestine, where your food gets ingested.

Because of oral resilience, the GALT doesn't react to most foods you eat as remote invaders. That is the reason you don't mount an immune system response to everything you eat. Nonetheless, the GALT is a similar part of the immune system that blows up to food and intercedes the hyperreactive immune response in food allergies, where the food is viewed as an invader.

The intestines likewise offer a place of refuge for helpful bacteria, which help in digestion and involve prime land so other harmful microorganisms can't move in. Dysbiosis is an imbalance of good and terrible bacteria in the gut. Because a significant number of its indications appear to be common reactions to certain foods, numerous people disregard the condition. Be that as it may, whenever left untreated, it can transform into the leaky gut syndrome, a significant cause of disease.

A leaky gut syndrome is part of the component that contributes to inflammation in the gastrointestinal (GI) tract and, accordingly, the rest of the body. Inflammation in the intestines disturbs the tight junctions, the paste that holds the cells of the intestines together in an independent cylinder. Most molecules are too enormous to fit through these junctions, so the main way for them to get away from the intestines and enter the blood is to be carried through the intestinal cells, from one side to the next.

With inflammation, the junctions become "leaky" and let things, for example, enormous food particles and bacteria out into the rest of the body, where the immune system can attack them. Along these lines, leaky gut syndrome, otherwise called intestinal hyperpermeability, contributes to autoimmune issues, joint pains, and food allergies and sensitivities.

Treating Your Symptoms with Nutrition

A lot of ongoing research has gone to the connection between what people eat and how it influences their inflammation levels. Numerous foods, regular in many kitchens, advance inflammation, and others have a recognizable decreasing impact on inflammation and may counteract it inside and out.

In this section, we take a gander at foods that can cause discomfort and how they're connected to inflammation. We disclose to you how to restructure your diet long-term to keep up great wellbeing and assist you with avoiding sometimes-shrouded inward inflammation.

Creating a diet that works for you

Creating an anti-inflammatory diet dependent on the foods your body acknowledges most, helps you remain healthy while keeping up — or holding — vitality levels and guaranteeing you get an adequate stockpile of vitamins and minerals.

Sometimes you may feel gassy or enlarged or get a cerebral pain in the wake of eating, yet have you at any point halted to believe that it's a particular food that is causing those symptoms, and it likely causes similar symptoms each time you eat it?

Nobody's diet or menu works for everybody. Your needs are not quite the same as your neighbor's; they're distinctive still from those of the person who lives in the neighborhood. In case you're sensitive to dairy products, it's almost guaranteed that foods made with bovine milk won't top your list of foods to eat. People with celiac disease or gluten sensitivities won't eat a lot of bread or heated products.

The initial phase in fitting an anti-inflammatory diet is to determine which foods are beneficial for you — which ones don't cause you pain, swelling, gas, or different sentiments of discomfort. Peruse the list of poisonous foods to determine which foods to avoid and create a menu that helps your body and tastes great.

Eating right for long-term benefits

Inflammatory foods can create moment symptoms just as long-term impacts. What's the damage in the long term? Inflammatory foods can speed the maturing procedure, add to rheumatoid joint pain and other joint issues, and invigorate inflammation in an assortment of ways.

Knowing which foods are inflammatory can be as straightforward as remembering one dependable guideline: The less it would seem that it did initially, the more inflammatory it likely is. Whole grains, for example, bulgur, dark-colored rice, and oats, all look as though they do in the wild, complete with the germ and the whole grain part, so they're probably going to be alright.

Whole, common foods still contain many, if not all, of the vitamins and minerals they ought to have. Eating these foods is particularly important for people with chronic diseases, hereditary issues, chronic pressure, or metabolic issue. These conditions increment the requirement for the vitamins and minerals that lessen inflammation and help the body work appropriately.

Overdoing it — or treating yourself — is alright from time to time, yet you ought to avoid certain inflammatory foods. Foods to avoid incorporate high-omega-6 oils, for example, those produced using corn, safflower, sunflower, and cottonseed; inflammatory soaked fats from animal sources, as found in prepared meats like bologna and franks, trans fats, and refined sugars.

Finding some kind of harmony is similarly as important as knowing which foods to eat. Make sure you're getting the right measure of proteins, healthy fats, vitamins and minerals, and different nutrients.

Enhancing Your Diet with an Anti-Inflammation Lifestyle

Creating an anti-inflammation diet is more than changing the foods you eat; it's focusing on a change in the way of life to give you a more advantageous life. Here are two regions of change that go hand-in-hand with the anti-inflammation diet:

- Restocking your kitchen with anti-inflammatory foods;

- Relearning how to cook; in case you're partial to pan-fried foods or even battered vegetables cooked in oil, become acclimated to eating somewhat better.

Investigate a portion of your propensities or indecencies. Do you smoke? Drink? What amount of activity do you get every day? Those are three major regions in which change — quitting any pretense of smoking, decreasing the amount you drink, and expanding the amount you work out — can make a significant improvement.

Physical action helps with weight reduction and upkeep, makes your heart work more productively, keeps your blood pressure in normal ranges, and decreases pressure, the main consideration in inflammation. Constant pressure drains your body of the nutrients you require for your immune system to work appropriately. Begin with some reflection or

yoga and take up a cardio exercise to slow maturing
of the mind and develop your muscles and nerves.

HOW METABOLISM WORKS

Your digestive system is in excess of a basic cylinder through which food travels. Digestion begins in your mouth and proceeds through your esophagus, stomach, small intestines, and colon. Your liver and pancreas likewise participate by delivering enzymes and bile to encourage the breakdown of food. The principal objective of digestion is to sort the great from the terrible so your body can extract the nutrients you require and discharge what might be harmful. A lot occurs between the time you put food in your mouth and when the remaining squanders are disposed of in the toilet.

To understand what's not working correctly in your digestion, you need to realize how a healthy digestion functions. The digestion procedure is mind-boggling, so to more readily understand it, we should perceive what occurs after you eat an "adjusted" dinner of fat, protein, and carbohydrates. The three fundamental macronutrients from which your body extracts vitality are a stir-fry of vegetables and chicken presented with rice and cooked in vegetable oil. The vegetables give a tad of carbohydrate, particularly as fiber; the chicken is, for the most part, protein; rice is, for the most part, carbohydrate as starch; and the vegetable oil is 100-percent fat.

The digestion procedure starts before you even begin eating; contemplating eating and smelling appealing foods "primes" your body to digest. However, it's in your mouth; when you bite your food and mix it with spit, then the solid digestion process is truly started. By chewing properly, you break down your food and make it easier for your stomach and intestines to digest. Spit covers your food to make it easier to swallow. It additionally contains a chemical (amylase) that begins to break down the starches in the rice.

In the wake of swallowing, the food travels down the esophagus into your stomach. The stomach agitates the food for a brief period and mixes it with hydrochloric acid and enzymes that digest the protein (pepsin) of your chicken. The agitating activity and acidity of your stomach help to transform your feast into a glue that will be much easier to digest. Following a couple of hours, small measures of your now-puréed dinner are discharged bit by bit into the initial segment of your small intestines.

At the point when the stir-fry lands in your small intestines, its acidity triggers the arrival of bile from your gall bladder and digestive enzymes from your pancreas. Since the fat in the oil of your stir-fry doesn't mix with water, bile mixes with the fat to make it easier to digest in the water-based condition of your digestive tract.

Your pancreas produces enzymes that digest the protein of the chicken (protease), the starches of the rice (amylase), and the fat of the vegetable oil (lipase). The cells covering your small intestines, likewise, contribute by delivering enzymes that break the little pieces of chicken protein into amino acids (peptidases), and break down sugars, and not entirely digested starches (disaccharidases like lactase, sucrose, and maltase).

People don't have the enzymes important to digest fiber, so it makes its way unblemished to the colon. The amino acids of chicken protein, the sugars of carbohydrates in the rice and vegetables, the fatty acids from fats in the vegetable oils, like different vitamins and minerals, are ingested into your body. After being absorbed in your small intestine, these nutrients are coursed back into your bloodstream.

After your body has taken all the nutrients it needs from your meal, the leftovers, which resemble nothing like your stir-fry, enter your colon (large intestines). Whatever you were not able to digest from your vegetables (primarily fiber) is fermented by the bacteria that make up your gut flora, and most of the remaining liquid is reabsorbed to compact your stools and make them solid. Your colon then acts as a storing place for your stools for a few hours or even a few days in some cases. And you know how the story ends!

The Importance of Stomach Acid

You read that right: Stomach acid is essential. Many people believe stomach acid is bad and that too much of it causes heartburn and acid reflux, but this is generally not the case. The fact is, most people don't produce enough stomach acid, which is crucial for proper digestion. Ever heard someone say they can't stomach meat or that it sits like a rock in their stomach for hours? A lack of adequate stomach acid is likely the problem. As we get older, our stomach can lose its ability to produce enough hydrochloric acid. Low stomach acid, or hypochlorhydria, is not something you hear about often, but it's widespread and can contribute to many digestive problems. A lack of stomach acid can have severe consequences and can contribute to malnutrition, nutrient deficiencies, and gastrointestinal infections. Since stomach acid is one of your first lines of defense against invaders, not having enough can put you at risk of food poisoning or other infections from harmful parasites, bacteria, or viruses. Low stomach acid can also promote the overgrowth of bacteria or yeast in your small intestines. Three-quarters of adults over 60 have low stomach acid—and just a single dose of proton-pump inhibitors, the most commonly prescribed type of antacid medication, is enough to reduce stomach acid production by more than 90 percent.

NUTRIENT ABSORPTION

The first role of stomach acid is to activate the enzyme pepsin, which is responsible for starting to break down protein in your stomach. One study showed that a normal acidity level in your stomach (pH of 2.5) allows you to break down 75 percent of beef protein. Without enough stomach acid, you can't properly digest the protein you eat. If the pH of your stomach reaches 5 (remember that the higher the pH, the less acidic), as is often the case in people taking antacids, only 25 percent of beef protein can be broken down, according to the same study. Inadequate protein digestion can result in the development of deficiencies in amino acids, the building blocks of protein. These deficiencies can, in turn, impair your body's production of neurotransmitters, the chemical messengers that help your brain cells communicate, and can even lead to depression, forgetfulness, and other mental problems over time.

The acidity of the stomach contents entering your small intestines then triggers the release of the bile from the gallbladder, which is crucial for the digestion of fat and the assimilation of fat-soluble nutrients. Insufficient acidity in your stomach can also, therefore, result in malnutrition and deficiencies in omega-3 fatty acids and vitamins A, D, E, and K, as well as inadequate absorption of the antioxidants CoenzymeQ10 (CoQ10), lycopene, tocopherols, and alpha- and beta-carotene.

Stomach acid starts the cascade required for healthy digestion by enhancing all the other steps of the digestive process. In addition to its roles in protein and fat metabolism, hydrochloric acid is also crucial in absorbing many important vitamins and minerals. Studies have shown the importance of stomach acid for proper absorption of the minerals iron, calcium, and zinc, as well as vitamins B6, B9 (folate), and B12. It's probable that stomach acid also plays a role in the absorption of any nutrients that are bound to protein, such as vitamins A, E, B1 (thiamine), B2 (riboflavin), and B3 (niacin). However, studies haven't yet been conducted on the impact of stomach acid on the absorption of these nutrients.

INFECTION PREVENTION

One of the primary jobs of a low pH in the stomach is to anticipate infections. This is sometimes alluded to as the "stomach acid boundary" because it genuinely goes about as a hindrance against infections. Most bacteria, parasites, and different organisms can't get by in the acidic milieu of the stomach. If you need more stomach acid, you are bound to get tainted with Salmonella, Campylobacter, Cholera, Listeria, C. Difficile, Giardia, and other frightful bugs. Not having enough stomach acid can likewise bring about an excess of alleged "great" bacteria in your small intestines, a condition called small intestinal bacterial abundance (SIBO). Gut-accommodating bacteria are important; however, such a large number of them in the wrong spot can cause enormous digestive issues.

FOOD SENSITIVITIES

Many digestive symptoms are associated with food sensitivities, which can be due in part to inadequate levels of stomach acid. Do you know how researchers make mice allergic to certain foods for the purposes of their studies? One of the most popular methods involves giving the mice encapsulated proteins from dairy, nuts, or eggs. The capsule acts as a barrier and prevents the proteins from being broken down properly and digested by the acid in the mouse's stomach. The result? The proteins move virtually intact into the intestines, potentially triggering an allergic reaction or the development of food sensitivities. Proteins are not meant to appear undigested in your intestines. If they do, they can confuse your immune system and trigger unpleasant reactions.

And this doesn't happen only in mice. If the pH in your stomach isn't acidic enough, the pepsin in your stomach won't be able to do its job effectively. If you have low stomach acid, you won't be able to digest most of the protein you eat properly. Large molecules of incompletely digested protein will make their way into your intestines, carrying with them the potential to induce the development of food allergies, sensitivities, and intolerances. Because of this, antacid medications, which make your stomach less acidic, are associated with a higher risk of developing food intolerances. You need sufficient stomach acid to digest your food; incomplete digestion can cause significant problems for your digestive health.

CAUSES OF LOW STOMACH ACID

Antacids, years on a vegetarian diet, stress, and certain gastrointestinal infections (such as H. pylori) can all reduce normal stomach-acid secretion and alter the normal pH of your stomach, compromising your digestion and health. The most common symptoms of low stomach acid (hypochlorhydria) include:

- Acid reflux, heartburn, and gastroesophageal reflux disease (GERD);

- Frequent belching after eating;

- Indigestion or an upset stomach after a meal;

- Excessive feeling of fullness after eating;

- Flatulence and gas;

- Constipation or diarrhea;

- Intestinal infections (parasites, yeasts, candida, bacteria);

- Small intestinal bacterial overgrowth (SIBO);

- Undigested food in stools;

- Food sensitivities and intolerances;

- Nutrient deficiencies;

- Anemia.

Don't these symptoms sound strangely similar to IBS and other common digestive problems?

<u>TESTING</u>

Tests to check stomach-acid levels are not done routinely, but you can ask your doctor to get tested. The best test is the Heidelberg Stomach Acid Test. It's not cheap, averaging around US$350, and is unfortunately rarely covered by health insurance. Even if your doctor has diagnosed you with acid reflux or GERD, it's unlikely he or she will refer you for this test automatically. Request it if you want to know whether your problems are truly due to too much stomach acid. The results may surprise you.

Some people also resort to a home test to evaluate their stomach acid level: the baking soda test. The validity of this test is not supported by any studies or evidence, but it can be worth a try. All you have to do is mix one-quarter teaspoon (one milliliter) of baking soda in a small glass of cold water and drink it first thing in the morning before breakfast. Watch the clock and time how long it takes before you belch. If you belch within the first two or three minutes, you probably have enough stomach acid. If it takes between three and five minutes, your stomach-acid levels are probably low, and if it takes more than five minutes, you are likely to have deficient stomach-acid levels. It's best to repeat this test on at least three different mornings to average the results and get a better sense of your stomach acid levels.

If you have low stomach acid, you can supplement with betaine HCl to replace the acid your stomach doesn't produce or take digestive bitters to increase your stomach acid production. Achieving the right level of acidity in your stomach can make a difference in alleviating your digestive problems, improving nutrient absorption, preventing gastrointestinal infections, and reducing some of your food sensitivities.

The Gallbladder

Your gallbladder has the important role of storing the bile produced by your liver. This organ can reach the size of a small pear when full, but it flattens out entirely after squeezing out its bile following the ingestion of fat. Bile is crucial for adequately digesting and absorbing fat and fat-soluble nutrients. If your gallbladder has been removed, the bile will simply drip continuously from your liver into your small intestines, instead of being stored and dumped all at once when you eat fat.

Even though it's possible to live without a gallbladder, it's certainly not ideal. Missing this critical organ can worsen digestive issues by forcing you to eat a low-fat diet. Low-fat diets are, by definition, high in carbs, and many carb-containing foods such as grains, dairy, and fruit can cause bloating, abdominal pain, gas, diarrhea, or constipation.

A few studies even indicate that some types of gallbladder issues have an autoimmune component. Considering that many autoimmune diseases seem to be aggravated by gluten, your diet has a huge role to play in your digestive health, whether you still have your gallbladder or had it removed. If you have gallbladder issues, sticking to REAL food that is naturally free of gluten and other ingredients that can be inflammatory, irritating, or allergenic can help you get your problem under control.

If your gallbladder has already been removed, the approach proposed in this book may still be beneficial for you. However, a few tweaks may be needed to facilitate fat digestion (as explained in more detail later). Supplementing with ox bile or using fats that don't require bile to be digested, such as the medium-chain triglycerides found in coconut oil, are examples of things you can do to tolerate fat without a gallbladder better. Properly digesting fat is crucial for both your overall and digestive health.

<u>**Your Gut Flora**</u>

If you think you're alone in your fight against digestive problems, think again. A huge number of microorganisms forming your gut flora (gut microbiota) live in your intestines. Although your gut flora can change over time, you're pretty much stuck with it, for better or for worse. A healthy gut flora can help your digestion run smoothly, while an unbalanced gut flora (gut dysbiosis) can lead to many digestive issues and even negatively affect your overall health.

The number of bacteria living on your body and inside your gut is enormous: 100 trillion bacteria. That is the same as 100,000 billion: a 1 followed by 14 zeros! It would take you thousands of years to count up to that number (counting one digit per second, 24/7)! Your body holds 10 times more bacteria than it has human cells. You're outnumbered in your own body!

The composition of your gut flora can vary depending on your diet, lifestyle, and age, but at any given time, you're carrying the equivalent of three to four pounds of bacteria. Even 60 percent of the weight of your stools is bacteria! The bacteria that live in your gut can have a tremendous influence on your health. It's estimated that at least 800 species and 7,000 different strains of bacteria live in your intestines, but the majority of them have yet to be identified.

Most of the microorganisms residing in the gastrointestinal tract of healthy people are commensal (gut-friendly), which means that they don't typically harm you and can even contribute to optimal health. In exchange for providing them a safe environment to live in, gut-friendly bacteria protect you against infections from pathogenic (harmful) microorganisms, in addition to stimulating your immune system, metabolizing dietary carcinogens, synthesizing some vitamins, and helping you better digest your foods. Also, the good bacteria in your GI tract are able to produce short-chain fatty acids (SCFAs), especially if your diet is rich in vegetables and fruits. That, in turn, contributes to the health of cells of your gut lining and provides you with an additional source of energy.

WHY IS A HEALTHY GUT FLORA SO IMPORTANT?

- Promotes immunity;

- Prevents gastrointestinal infections;

- Reduces inflammation;

- Metabolizes dietary carcinogens and heavy metals;

- Synthesizes some nutrients (vitamins K and B12, biotin, short-chain fatty acids);

- Contributes to digestion;

- Regulates body weight;

- Protects the integrity of your gut lining.

Somewhere in the range of 70 and 80 percent of your immune system is situated in your gut. A healthy gut flora speaks with your immune system to assist it with separating great microorganisms from awful ones. That helps your body know which bacteria to wreck and which to ensure to keep up a healthy equalization in your intestines. On the off chance that your digestion isn't working appropriately, odds are your immune system isn't, either. A bumbling immune system not just puts you at a greater danger of becoming ill, yet it additionally improves your probability of creating food sensitivities and autoimmune disorders. Your gut vegetation likewise ensures the honesty of the intestinal coating to avert irregular intestinal penetrability (known as leaky gut), which can prompt further food prejudices and add to the improvement or compounding of autoimmune disorders.

GUT DYSBIOSIS IS ASSOCIATED WITH:

- IBS;

- Celiac disease;

- Inflammatory bowel disorders (Crohn's disease and ulcerative colitis);

- GERD;

- Some cancers;

- Obesity;

- Allergies and food sensitivities;

- Heart diseases;

- Mental disorders (autism, schizophrenia, anxiety, depression);

- And many more.

Many factors can influence your gut flora over the course of your life. Your digestive tract was completely sterile until birth, when it was colonized either by the bacteria from your mother's flora if you were born naturally or from any bacteria in your environment if you were born via C-section. The foods you eat throughout your life, infections, and the use of medications, especially antibiotics, can all drastically alter your gut flora balance. Studies show that a single course of antibiotics can result in a loss of the biodiversity of your gut flora within three to four days. Although your gut flora can slowly start to restore itself once you discontinue your antibiotics, researchers have shown that it usually never returns fully to its initial composition. Table 4 lists many factors that can affect your gut flora positively or negatively. In the next chapters, you will learn how you can try to improve your gut flora to optimize your digestion, reduce food sensitivities, and improve your overall health by choosing the right foods (including fermented foods) and using probiotic supplements.

The Gut-Brain Axis

Your gastrointestinal system is the oldest and most evolved organ in your body. It is a fact that there are more nerve tissues in your digestive system than in your brain. The nerve system in your gastrointestinal tract is so complex that it's the only organ that can work completely independently of the brain. This complex system, and its impact on your brain and body, is often referred to as the brain-gut axis. From regulating your food intake to the metabolism of glucose and fat, bone metabolism, and mental health, the gut-brain axis appears to play many important roles, many of which have yet to be elucidated.

Even though the gut-brain axis is extremely complex, you've probably already experienced the strong connection between your gut and your brain in your personal life. Have you ever noticed that stress could affect your bowel movements? Or had butterflies in your stomach before speaking in public? Perhaps you've sometimes just had a gut feeling about something. It's no coincidence that emotions and feelings often seem to be connected with our digestive system.

There is a strong connection between our brain and intestines, and it works both ways. Stress can harm your gut flora and even damage your intestines while bloating and problems with bowel movements can result in depression, anxiety, and other mental disorders. In fact, 50 to 90 percent of people with IBS report experiencing one of these mental conditions.

This might be due, in part, to the altered serotonin levels found in the guts of people with digestive issues. Serotonin is an important neurotransmitter found in your brain that helps you feel happy, calm, and relaxed. What many people don't know, however, is that 95 percent of the serotonin in your body is found in your GI tract. The serotonin in your gut influences the communication between your gut and your brain and affects intestinal motility, fluid secretion in your digestive system, and the sensation of pain in your abdomen. People with IBS have abnormal serotonin levels in their gut, which further reinforces the importance of the gut-brain axis.

Chapter 7 addresses the mind-body connection because you can't expect to improve your digestive health without also taking care of your mind.

Intestinal Permeability: When Your Gut Goes Leaky

Your intestines constitute an important barrier — and the largest one — between your body and the environment. The surface of your small intestines is so big that it corresponds to 100 times the surface area of your skin. Like your skin, your intestines have the role of protecting you against invaders like harmful microorganisms and toxins.

Did you know that what's inside your digestive system is outside your body? It's when nutrients are absorbed and circulated in your bloodstream that they truly enter your body. One of the roles of your digestive system is to meticulously sort the good from the bad in the food you eat, making sure that only the beneficial stuff, such as nutrients, enters the body, and keeping out bacteria, toxins, and waste products until they can be flushed away.

Your gut lining is made of a single layer of epithelial cells that are, amazingly, all that keeps what's in your intestines from reaching your bloodstream. This microscopic cellular barrier is all that separates you from the outside world. It sticks together with the help of what are called tight junctions. Tight junctions form connections like "holding hands" to build your gut lining, opening when necessary to let in nutrients.

If your intestinal lining is compromised, some of the cells lining your gut can become too weak to hold hands. Some of the tight junctions can break, allowing incompletely digested nutrients, toxins, and bacteria to enter your bloodstream. When this happens, it's called increased intestinal permeability, or leaky gut.

ANTI-INFLAMMATORY HERBS AND NATURAL SOURCES

The idea of anti-inflammatory herbs is an interesting one in the world of naturopathy and everyday wellbeing. The motivation behind why I float towards them is because, in the domain of inflammation and anti-inflammatory diets, they're a nice middle ground. A few people require an absolute anti-inflammatory diet, eating just foods that promote the suppressing of inflammation in the body. Others are on the Standard American Diet, eating a large group of foods that are known to cause inflammation in the body and bother numerous disorders and conditions. Anti-inflammatory herbs are nicely in the middle. Foods, in general, are said to be either pro-inflammatory or anti-inflammatory. As you would have speculated, foods that are pro-inflammatory will increase the measure of inflammation happening in various parts of your body, will increase the pain related to it, and may likewise enhance your risk of having a chronic disease. Pro-inflammatory foods are mostly lousy nourishments, sugars, fast foods, exceptionally processed foods, and meats high in fat.

In any case, that appears to be a bit over the top. That is the reason I love the possibility of anti-inflammatory herbs. They're an excellent middle ground in the world of inflammation, allowing you to remain healthy in that field without placing an over the top spotlight on inflammation in general. Normally, eating some form of regular anti-inflammatory foods is key because it helps diminish the risk of things like arthritis and chronic autoimmune diseases. Also, because of the way that natural creations are generally genuinely solid, anti-inflammatory herbs are a great expansion to dinners, just as in supplements.

Herbs generally have a wide assortment of medical advantages, and because inflammation is a to some degree complex process in the body, herbs can influence inflammation in various ways. Inflammation, when conveyed past sensible points of confinement, can turn into a kind of autoimmune condition. It starts as negative boosts cause white blood cells to enact to protect the region being contrarily influenced. Inflammation is vital to the mending process. However, chronic inflammation can cause lots of long-term problems and is frequently extreme, similar to an unfavorably susceptible response.

Here are probably the best, most dominant anti-inflammatory herbs:

1. Turmeric. Turmeric is a spice typical to most Indian foods. In spite of the fact that it has numerous other medicinal benefits, turmeric is a ground-breaking anti-inflammatory herb. Be that as it may, it takes a bit of time to begin working, so if you don't care for the flavor of turmeric, you should consider taking it in container form.

2. Ginger. Ginger is likewise a spice that is utilized frequently in Asian cooking. This spice also has a strong flavor and takes a bit of time to produce results inside the body. Ginger is exceptionally adaptable, being

utilized in a range of the two foods and drinks, so filling your diet with it shouldn't be an over the top test. You can drink ginger tea, ginger beer, utilize ginger in baked goods, and spice meats with it.

3. Omega 3 Essential Fatty Acids. Although these aren't herbs, omega 3 basic fatty acids are something that everybody needs a higher amount of in their diets. They're not just anti-inflammatory, they have a range of other medicinal benefits the whole way across the body.

4. Licorice. Licorice is another herb that is compelling in the world of anti-inflammation. It's a great herb to take because of its decent variety. Licorice is helpful because it very well may be added to pretty much anything, similar to treat, tea, baked goods, vegetables, meats, and that's only the tip of the iceberg, making it simple to get a great everyday portion.

5. Mangosteen Juice. Mangosteen is an organic product local to Asia that has amazing anti-inflammatory properties. Mangosteen juice is turning out to be increasingly more mainstream with persons who are experiencing the pain of arthritis, and it even has a good flavor. Numerous people substitute it for orange juice in their morning breakfast.

DETERMINING INFLAMMATION'S ROLE IN CHRONIC DISEASES

The body is equipped to take care of itself in many situations, sending signals to create healthy inflammation levels where needed. Catch a cold, and the immune system instantly sends a message to the body to start fighting it off. Twist your ankle while hiking, and the area around it instantly starts to swell, creating a cushioned protection while the injury begins to heal.

Sometimes, however, the body's defense mechanism works against itself, creating problems instead of solving them. Whether the signals get crossed, or the process kicks into high gear, the body may fight itself when there's no real reason to engage. The result of this overreaction is a chronic illness. That could impact the heart, the nerves, the lungs, the joints — just about any organ and tissue.

In this chapter, we will look at a variety of chronic illnesses, from heart disease, asthma, and diabetes to obesity and problems with the digestive and immune systems. In addition to helping you gain a better understanding of these illnesses, we will identify the role inflammation plays in each of them as well as what you can do to prevent or delay symptoms.

Understanding Chronic Diseases

Chronic diseases are those that aren't transmittable; that is, they're not infectious. They're generally long-enduring and don't simply leave alone like a cold or this season's flu virus does. Chronic diseases incorporate heart disease, diabetes, cancer, and arthritis — all diseases that attack the body and plan to remain. Most chronic diseases are never relieved totally, so your most logical option is to avoid getting them in any case.

The Centers for Disease Control offer some interesting — and frightening — insights concerning chronic diseases:

- Chronic diseases are answerable for 7 of 10 deaths in the United States every year.

- About 133 million Americans — a large portion of the grown-ups — live with at least one form of chronic illness.

- More than 75 percent of medicinal services expenses can be credited to chronic disease.

Inflammation is a common denominator among chronic diseases. Causes of inflammation — for example, an inflammatory diet, cigarette smoking, chronic infections, day by day stress, supplement inadequacies, poisons, and absence of activity — joined with hereditary inclinations are a formula for chronic disease.

These factors can lead to systemic inflammation, which can later lead to chronic diseases, for example, heart and cardiovascular diseases, metabolic disorders (diabetes, obesity, metabolic syndrome), bone disease, and gloom. Inflammation leads to low vitality and makes you increasingly prone to becoming ill and irritable, making you less propelled to practice and further leading to skeletal muscle shortcoming and more inflammation.

This cycle is self-sustaining — except if you begin to take care of business by changing your diet and lifestyle. Research has shown that dietary and lifestyle changes are more successful than any prescription in decreasing your risk of chronic disease and can anticipate prediabetes from transforming into diabetes. Remember that changing your diet to stop inflammation isn't only a transitory fix — it's something you need to focus on following for a mind-blowing rest.

Inflammation might be a fundamental cause in various disease processes because it meddles with numerous body capacities. For instance, the leaky gut syndrome is a part of the system by which food allergies, sensitivities, prejudices, and poisons assume a job in the improvement of autoimmune diseases.

Autoimmune diseases are chronic diseases in which the body attacks itself all through of-control inflammation. Other than hereditary qualities, dietary factors assume a significant job in autoimmune diseases. For instance, examines have shown that people with specific types of autoimmune diseases, for example, Sjögren's syndrome and Graves' disease, have a greater narrow mindedness to gluten and a higher risk of creating celiac disease.

Interfacing Heart Disease, Obesity, and Diabetes to Inflammation

Your body frequently doesn't take on each disease in turn. Rather, you may get one chronic illness at first, and that illness can lead to other issues. Obesity, for instance, is viewed as a chronic disease all alone, but at the same time, it's a factor in other chronic illnesses, for example, heart disease and diabetes. You can decrease your risk for every one of these illnesses by removing inflammatory foods and factors from your lifestyle.

In this section, we discuss the role inflammation plays in creating heart disease, obesity, and diabetes.

Heart disease: Affecting heart work

Clinical research has revealed a serious connection between inflammation and heart disease, the leading cause of death for the people in the United States. Inflammation assumes a relevant role in atherosclerosis, wherein fatty stores develop in the coating of the courses.

At the point when inflammation damages blood vessels, the body utilizes cholesterol to fix them up, creating plaque that can lead to atherosclerosis and other heart-related diseases. (See the close by sidebar for subtleties.)

The association between inflammation and heart disease is certain. The certainty is, to such an extent, that in 2003 the American Heart Association (AHA) and the Centers for Disease Control and Prevention (CDC) gave a joint restorative articulation opening the entryway for the utilization of inflammatory markers. For example, the C-reactive protein in the blood is diagnosing heart disease and checking its seriousness. The two associations ended, giving the alright to specialists to begin drawing a line interfacing inflammation to heart disease.

In this section, we discuss common types of heart disease related to inflammation and examine a couple of ways to lower your risk factors.

Seeing common types of heart disease

The types of heart disease range from a minor arrhythmia — irregular heart-beat — to a significant heart attack or stroke. Symptoms and causes shift, yet everyone conveys its very own risk factors, treatment, and, by and large, preventive measures to avoid it through and through. Here we investigate the most common types of heart disease related to inflammation and signs you can search for to distinguish everyone:

- Cardiovascular disease: Cardiovascular disease, or atherosclerosis, is commonly known as hardening of the arteries. Cardiovascular disease is caused by a buildup of fatty plaques in your arteries, which, over time, can make your arteries hard and stiff.

- Major risk factors of cardiovascular disease are smoking, being overweight, lack of exercise, and an unhealthy diet.

- Coronary artery disease: Coronary artery disease (CAD) occurs when fatty plaque builds up in the arteries of the heart, and the CDC lists it as the most common form of heart disease in the United States. More than 7 million Americans have coronary artery disease, and an estimated 500,000 Americans die from it each year.

The plaque buildup can lead to angina or chest pain that occurs when the heart doesn't receive enough blood, which can later lead to more severe problems such as heart failure, arrhythmia, or heart attack. Signs of coronary artery disease include chest pain or discomfort, shortness of breath, pain in the arms or shoulder, feeling lightheaded or faint, or pain in the jaw, neck, or back.

Reducing your risk factors for heart disease

The American Heart Association reports that in 2006, approximately 73,600,000 people had high blood pressure, and 17,600,000 had coronary artery disease. Cardiovascular disease caused the deaths of more than 831,200 people in 2006, accounting for more than 34 percent of all deaths that year.

Understanding what those numbers mean and how they relate to you is an essential step in taking away the fear of numbers while you tailor your lifestyle to keep you from being a statistic. The best way to do that is to look at the risk factors, compare them to your lifestyle, and make changes to reduce the risks you can control.

Obesity: Adding extra pounds

Although many industrialized countries have seen steady increases in the rates of obesity, none have seen as big a boost as the United States: In a ten-year period, from 1997 to 2007, the percentage of obese people in the U.S. climbed from 19.4 percent to 26.6 percent.

Blaming the fast-food industry, lack of exercise, or a general diet of overindulgence for the world's expanding waistline is easy, but there are hidden explanations as well. Researchers are finding more and more instances in which inflammation seems not only to prevent weight loss but also to cause people to gain even more weight.

Obesity puts the body into a state of chronic, low-grade inflammation, which is born in the fat cells lying under the skin. When a body is obese, it secretes chemicals called cytokines from the glial cells, which are part of the nervous system. These cytokines are molecules that set inflammation into motion.

Some of them, interleukin-1 (IL-1) and TFN-alpha can make you sleepy and irritable. These molecules alert the liver to act immediately, and the liver creates C-reactive protein, which is one sign of inflammation.

White adipose tissue, or fat cells, release several inflammatory chemical signals, called adipokines, that affect the body as a whole. The fat cells then become part of the endocrine system — the system that regulates growth and reproduction and, when out of balance, increases the risk of insulin resistance, diabetes, heart disease, and other illnesses.

How cortisol discharge because of stress and promotes weight gain

At the point when your body is under stress, or your blood contains low degrees of hormones called glucocorticoids, the pituitary organ in the cerebrum secretes a hormone called acetylcholinesterase (ACTH) which signals the adrenal organ on the kidney to emit cortisol. Cortisol is a hormone that increases blood sugar, stifles the immune system, diminishes bone formation, and influences fat, protein, and carbohydrate digestion, which can lead to weight gain. Cortisol levels are controlled by the part of the mind called the nerve center.

The low-level chronic inflammation of obesity makes your mind and body less responsive to the typical prompts (intervened by the adipokines) that sign when you're full and help you to keep up healthy body weight. The inflammation additionally advises your adrenal organs to produce a higher amount of the compound cortisol.

Cortisol is your body's natural anti-inflammatory chemical and is produced in high sums during chronic stress and obesity. Cortisol helps keep vitality on track by deciding the right sort and measure of carbohydrate, fat, or protein that your body needs at a particular time. It moves the body's fat stores starting with one area, then onto the next, and averts the arrival of substances in the body that leads to inflammation.

Cortisol's response to inflammation is to produce increasingly fat cells around the stomach area (midsection fat). Which at that point, increases liquid maintenance, raises blood pressure, increases blood sugar, and the risk of insulin opposition, and increases the risks of memory misfortune and muscle and bone shortcoming.

Diabetes: Wreaking ruin with your blood sugar

Inflammation and blood sugar have a fairly turbulent, roundabout relationship. At the point when you have high blood sugar, chemicals are discharged all through your body, weakening your immune system and getting inflammation is going to help protect the body. Because the immune system has been debilitated, in any case, inflammation goes into overdrive and raises the blood sugar, further weakening the immune system.

At the point when you eat, your body breaks down carbohydrates into glucose, a straightforward sugar that travels through your blood and that your muscle cells and different cells take in and use as a vitality source. Insulin fills in as the glucose police in that it controls how much glucose remains in your blood. At the point when glucose starts to develop, the pancreas (the organ behind the stomach) discharges more insulin.

In the perfect circumstance, the pancreas produces the insulin the body needs, and the body cells react by taking in sugar. Be that as it may, a condition called insulin obstruction inhibits the way glucose can get into the body's cells. Inflammation might be behind the poor gathering between the cells and the insulin signals. The glucose develops in the blood, leading to promote inflammation and heightening the problem.

Inflammation from various causes increases insulin opposition because the cells become less responsive to the job of insulin in attempting to get the glucose into the cell. In like manner, high blood sugar levels caused by eating an excessive number of desserts, void calories, and basically carbohydrates force the pancreas to produce more insulin to attempt to tidy up the glucose and carry it into the cells. The more you charge your pancreas by eating sugary foods, the almost certain your cells will become insulin safe, expanding your risk for diabetes.

Infection, stress, poisons, hereditary factors, and less than stellar eating routine increase inflammation, which contributes to increased insulin obstruction. Insulin opposition leads to diminished glucose digestion, which leads to high blood sugar and high insulin levels. High blood sugar and insulin levels add to weight gain and increased (fat) tissue. High blood sugar, insulin levels, and terrible fats add to advance inflammation by blocking delta-6 desaturase, a protein that is important in diminishing inflammation, and upgrading delta-5, an inflammatory chemical.

The way to halting the cycle is to discover ways to lower the inflammation, which at that point attempts to lower the blood sugar levels.

Contributing to Cancer

Researchers continue to find connections between cancer and inflammation.

For example, medical researchers have found that

- Inflammation can cause DNA changes. A study conducted by the Massachusetts Institute of Technology (MIT) shows a correlation between the DNA damage caused by inflammation and colorectal cancer.

- Recurring infections due to viruses, bacteria, and even overgrowth of yeast can set the body up, so it's prone to developing cancer cells. For example, certain strains of HPV (human papillomavirus) increase the risk of developing cervical cancer.

- Toxins in food, like nitrosamines in cured and smoked meats, can stimulate the growth of cancer cells.

- Chronic inflammation helps existing tumors grow and can encourage cancer stem cells to replicate. Research at the University of Michigan's Comprehensive Cancer Center in 2010 suggested that the link between the stem cells of breast cancer and inflammation can promote the recurrence of cancer.

When inflammation persists, it creates a negative environment that can support the development of tumors, and pre-cancerous cells can become malignant. Researchers believe this happens because many of the processes that occur in chronic inflammation can contribute to tumor growth and disease progression.

Inflammation starts with the help of cytokines — chemicals that send signals to specific cells to either enhance or suppress the body's immune system. These cytokines are proteins whose primary responsibility is to attack foreign bodies or damaged cells or to signal other parts of the immune system to get in gear and attack. Cancer cells are just the type of cells cytokines should be attacking. However, although cancer cells have somehow lost their ability to control their growth, they're otherwise normal, healthy cells. Because of this, the immune system doesn't recognize these cells as foreign, so it doesn't attack.

Asthma: Inflaming the Lungs

Inflammation plays an important role in the everyday functioning of the lungs. Think of all the bacteria, viruses, dust, and everything else floating through the air, and then think of yourself breathing it in. Small amounts of inflammation are at work throughout the day battling these particles, creating and using an antibody called immunoglobulin E (IgE) to aid in breaking down the pollutants.

The lungs of people with asthma, however, overreact to these particles. The immune system mass-produces the IgE antibodies, which then attach to something called mast cells. Each time someone with asthma inhales the offending particles, the antibodies lock onto the invaders and cause the mast cells to release histamine and leukotrienes, which irritate the lining of the airways. The irritation causes the airways to spasm and constrict, making breathing difficult; the harder the person tries to breathe, the more irritated and constricted the airways become.

Atopy, or IgE reactions, is the most significant predisposing factor for developing asthma. Many people with asthma also have a sensitivity to sulfites, which are found in certain foods and are used in wine-making and preserving dried fruit.

Asthma can be caused by a variety of factors that result in airway inflammation, and triggers for asthma attacks may be allergic or nonallergic. Allergic asthma, or extrinsic asthma, is triggered by allergens. Nonallergic asthma, or intrinsic asthma, can be triggered by anything but is not considered an allergic reaction.

Allergic triggers include the following:

- Cat or dog hair and saliva;

- Dust mites, mold, or spores;

- Pollen.

Non-allergic triggers include the following:

- Smoke, smog, fumes;

- Natural gas, cooking fuel;

- Exercise;

- Viral respiratory infections;

- Weather changes, such as exposure to cold air.

Disrupting Your Digestive System

Inflammation steps in when the digestive tract goes cockeyed. Regardless of whether it is because something has physically harmed the tract, or you've eaten your way to inconvenience. Sometimes the inflammation takes the form of a gentle stomach issue, for example, diarrhea or obstruction, and different times it can lead to something considerably more genuine.

Crohn's disease and ulcerative colitis are forms of inflammatory entrail disease (IBD), which are inflammation-related diseases that influence the colon and small intestines. In the two conditions, parts of the digestive tract — otherwise called the gastrointestinal (GI) tract — become inflamed and create problems with digestion:

- Crohn's disease: Crohn's disease causes inflammation anyplace along the GI tract and can spread into the layers of gut tissue. It can cause inflammation in a few zones of the intestinal tract on the double, leaving healthy inside caught between two portions of diseased entrail.

- Specialists trust Crohn's disease is an aftereffect of the body's immune system. The immune system creates an inflammatory response to misidentified invaders, assembling a protective region against specific foods. What results is abdominal pain and diarrhea as the body endeavors to free itself of the invaders. Different symptoms of Crohn's disease incorporate rectal dying, weight loss, fatigue, skin aggravations, and fever. Draining can get over the top, leading to weakness (low iron).

- Ulcerative colitis: Ulcerative colitis creates inflammation and ulcers just in the top layer of the covering of the digestive organ, and it frequently influences the rectum. Symptoms of ulcerative colitis are fundamentally the same as those of Crohn's disease, causing some disarray in attempting to build up a diagnose between the two. The symptoms incorporate iron deficiency, fatigue, weight loss, loss of hunger, bloody diarrhea mixed with bodily fluid, loss of body liquids and nutrients, skin sores, joint pain and hindered development (particularly in kids), and abdominal pain.

Prescriptions can ease a portion of the discomfort of inside inflammatory disorders, and medical procedure is crucial for around 66% of people with Crohn's disease.

Inflammation of the digestive tract can cause further problems in different parts of the body as well. The leaky gut syndrome is a marvel whereby the cells of the gastrointestinal tract are inflamed and never again provide a protective obstruction between within and outside worlds of your digestive tract. It likewise can make you feel enlarged and fatigued, particularly in the wake of eating.

The initial step to treating IBD is to distinguish the causes of inflammation — diet, stressors, supplement lacks, hereditary powerlessness, etc. Next, expel the inflammatory foods from your diet. You additionally need to recuperate the gut, which may include taking anti-inflammatory medications and enhancements, for example, omega-3 fatty acids and l-glutamine. The inflamed gut can't retain vitamins, for example, B12, so in the wake of recuperating, you would then be able to address supplement inadequacies.

Thumping Your Immune System Off-kilter

The body's immune system is a brilliant thing when it's working correctly. It keeps infection under control and protects a harmed territory from getting reinjured while it recuperates. Sometimes, be that as it may, the immune system fizzles and conveys signals when none are required. In those occurrences, the inflammation attacks the body, creating autoimmune disorders, for example, lupus, rheumatoid arthritis, and numerous sclerosis. We discuss these autoimmune disorders in this section.

Autoimmune disorders appear to be related to leaky gut syndrome (see the first section), and people with these disorders likewise have a higher frequency of nutrient D lack. An anti-inflammatory diet and stress decrease may improve autoimmune conditions.

Getting to know lupus

The systemic lupus erythematosus (SLE) is an autoimmune disorder that affects the kidneys and other organs, as well as the skin and joints.

Lupus appears to be a women's disease for the most part — more than 90 percent of those diagnosed are women between the ages of 15 and 40. People with relatives who have lupus have a 5 to 13 percent chance of developing the disease, although people whose mothers have lupus have just a 5 percent chance of getting it. In most cases, people diagnosed with lupus have a relative who has been diagnosed with some other autoimmune disease.

Although lupus is mostly a genetic disorder, some environmental factors can trigger the illness: exposure to ultraviolet sun rays or rays from fluorescent bulbs, sulfa drugs, penicillin, an infection, a cold or other viral infection, exhaustion, stress, or an injury.

The severity of SLE can range widely; it can be very mild, or it can turn fatal.

Symptoms of SLE vary according to which part of the body is affected:

- Brain and nervous system: Symptoms may include headaches, personality changes, psychotic episodes, tingling in the arms and legs, and seizures.

- Digestive tract: Symptoms may include nausea, vomiting, and abdominal pain.

- Kidneys: Look for discolored urine.

- Heart: Symptoms include arrhythmia.

- Lungs: Symptoms include coughing up blood.

- Skin: Skin rashes, particularly on the face, appear if SLE is affecting the skin.

Some common symptoms, regardless of where SLE attacks, are fatigue, weight loss, unexplained fever, sores in the mouth, and hair loss.

There's no cure for SLE, but you can control the symptoms. Dietary changes are one way to help relieve some of the pain and discomfort. Some medications alleviate discomfort for some varieties of SLE, and corticosteroid creams are used for skin rashes.

Arthritis: Making your joints ache

The word arthritis literally means "inflammation of the joints." Most forms of arthritis are autoimmune diseases, a result of a misinformed attack by the immune system on different parts of the body. Some of the more well-known forms of arthritis caused by inflammation are:

- Rheumatoid arthritis;

- Gout;

- Systemic lupus erythematosus;

- Degenerative joint disease.

Some of the symptoms of inflammation associated with arthritis are redness, joint pain, warm swollen areas, and limited ability to bend the joints.

Research has shown that certain foods, such as those in the nightshade or Solanaceae family (potatoes, tomatoes, eggplant, bell peppers), contribute to inflammation in rheumatoid arthritis (RA) and osteoarthritis (OA) for some people. About 10 percent of people have sensitivities or allergies to the nightshade family, and, as with any sensitivity, this situation can increase the risk of arthritis. Anti-inflammatory foods such as fish oil help reduce the inflammation of RA and OA.

Looking at osteoarthritis

In osteoarthritis, inflammation of the joint compresses the nerves and causes the shock-absorbing system between the joints to degenerate. Osteoarthritis is also known as age-related arthritis, and with good reason: It affects more than 70 percent of adults between the ages of 55 and 78. The majority of those affected are women.

Osteoarthritis may also be caused by obesity or long-term overuse of a joint during work or in sports. Repeated motion and injuries contribute to the inflammatory process in arthritis. For example, a football player who injures himself is more susceptible to arthritis in the affected area. A joint injury at a younger age can mean osteoarthritis later.

Although osteoarthritis isn't curable, you can manage its pain and other symptoms. Some doctors advise taking acetaminophen for pain, and lifestyle changes may also relieve some of the tenderness. Exercise helps keep the joints moving and can help with weight loss, mainly if that's relevant to osteoarthritis.

Experts also recommend getting plenty of rest, keeping the joints protected, and eating a healthy, well-balanced diet. Part of that includes drinking enough water to keep the joints and the rest of the body hydrated.

Recognizing rheumatoid arthritis

Rheumatoid arthritis (RA) is an autoimmune disease that causes inflammation in the lining of the smaller joints in the hands and feet, often leading to bone deterioration and joint deformity. Some sufferers experience intermittent flare-ups, and others see the symptoms and pain go into a remission-like dormancy for long periods.

More than 1.3 million Americans suffer from RA — about 1 percent of the country's population. It occurs two or three times as often in women as it does in men and generally occurs between the ages of 30 and 60, although it can occur in teens and even children.

No one knows the cause of RA, although researchers have a list of suspects. Some believe an infectious bacteria or virus triggers it, and others think it may be linked to a female hormone, resulting in the high differential between the number of women who develop RA over men. Many researchers believe smoking plays a role as well, at least by weakening the body's immune system.

Diagnosis includes checking for inflammation in the blood with tests such as the C-reactive protein (CRP) test and radiological studies. Approximately 75 percent of people test positive for the rheumatoid factor (RF) antibody in their blood, which may be a sign of RA. Having RF show up on a blood test doesn't necessarily mean you have it, nor does not having RF say you don't, because about 20 percent of tests result in false positives and false negatives. Your doctor will take into account your clinical symptoms combined with these tests to determine your diagnosis.

Rheumatoid arthritis is a chronic disease, but it's manageable. Doctors may prescribe certain medications to relieve the pain of rheumatoid arthritis, but people with RA can also do many things at home without a prescription. Applying heat and cold to the affected area can alleviate some of the pain, and exercising regularly helps keep bones and joints moving, reducing the risk of stiffness.

Following an anti-inflammatory diet and avoiding the nightshade family can aid in reducing the pain and inflammation of RA. Tobacco is also in the nightshade family, so avoid smoking as well.

Nerve attacks: Linking inflammation to multiple sclerosis

Multiple sclerosis (MS) is an autoimmune disorder that showcases how violent the human body can be when it turns on itself. With multiple sclerosis, the body's immune system eats away at the protective covering that envelops the nerves, interfering with communication between the nerves and the brain and eventually leading to a degeneration of the nerves themselves. The process MS follows is irreversible. There's no cure, but treatment can lessen the severity of the attacks.

Multiple sclerosis may be challenging to diagnose in the early stages because symptoms tend to come and go, often not resurfacing for months. Symptoms also vary greatly; they may include numbness or tingling in the arms and legs, partial or complete loss of vision, double vision or blurred vision, fatigue, dizziness, and electric shock-type sensations that occur when the head moves in a certain way. In the most severe cases, people lose the ability to walk or talk.

MS tends to occur in women twice as often as in men, and it's typically diagnosed in people between the ages of 20 and 40. If a member of your family has MS, you have a 1 to 3 percent chance of inheriting the disease. Caucasians whose families originated in northern Europe are at higher risk.

Here are several things you can do at home to relieve the symptoms of multiple sclerosis:

- Cool down. Multiple sclerosis symptoms tend to flare up when your body temperature rises. Try taking a cool bath to bring your temperature back down.

- Get plenty of rest. Fatigue is a common symptom and getting rest can help you feel better.

- Exercise. Keeping active with mild aerobic exercise helps build strength and muscle coordination if you have mild to moderate MS.

- Watch your diet. Researchers believe multiple sclerosis is an autoimmune disorder caused by inflammation, so look for anti-inflammatory foods.

ANTI-INFLAMMATORY HERBS AND SUPPLEMENTS

Changing your diet to include anti-inflammatory foods, spices, herbs, and beverages is the first and most important step in the battle against inflammation and chronic disease. Getting a lot of good exercises — both heart-pumping cardiovascular workouts and relaxing yoga — is another good step.

Finding those supplements — natural herbs and enzymes — that give your new diet that extra boost is a bonus in the fight against inflammation. From herbs that keep migraines at bay to vitamins that help reduce the risk of cancer, supplements should be part of your daily routine. We discuss our top ten anti-inflammatory herbs and supplement picks in this chapter. Read on for info on the benefits, the recommended dosages, and the cautions and contraindications associated with these supplements.

Always consult a physician or pharmacist who is knowledgeable in herbs, supplements, and their interactions before trying any herbs or supplements on your own.

Omega-3 Fatty Acids: Mixed EPA and DHA from Fish Oils

Eicosapentaenoic acid (EPA) and docosahexaenoic acid (DHA) are two essential fatty acids derived from fish and some vegetarian sources. You can't make these fatty acids in your body — that's why they're essential fatty acids — so you need to get them from food or supplements daily. EPA and DHA are anti-inflammatory superstars. They compete against a pro-inflammatory compound called arachidonic acid (AA), avoiding their incorporation into cellular membranes.

Use fish (such as salmon and sardines) and fish oils as your primary sources of EPA and DHA. Vegetarian sources of omega-3 fatty acids (flax and chia, for example) contain alpha-linolenic acid (ALA), which gets converted into EPA.

If you can't find fish that are low in mercury and other toxins, take a high-quality fish oil supplement with both EPA and DHA for an anti-inflammatory diet.

Just as important as the positives that take place when you do supplement your diet with fish oils is what happens when you don't: Some studies have linked an omega-3 deficiency to an increased risk of depression.

Here are some basic ideas you should know about increasing your intake of mixed EPA and DHA from fish oils:

- Checking for quality: Choose fish oil supplements that are good manufacturing practice (GMP) -certified and tested for heavy metals. They should smell like fresh fish when you bite into a capsule. Quality fish oils cost a little more than other brands and have been tested for shelf stability.

- Dosing: Take 1 to 4 grams daily of a mixed EPA/DHA.

- Cautions/contraindications: Because fish oils have benefits similar to blood thinners, they may increase the effect of pharmaceutical blood thinners, such as warfarin (Coumadin).

Ginger

The root of the ginger plant has increased in popularity in recent years, and no wonder — it has multiple anti-inflammatory benefits and helps reduce symptoms in inflammatory disorders. Among the benefits of ginger, and more specifically gingerroot, are the following:

It decreases inflammation by inhibiting the cyclooxygenase and lipoxygenase pathways, prostaglandin E2, thromboxane B2, and tumor necrosis factor (TNF-alpha).

- It reduces pain in disorders such as osteoarthritis and rheumatoid arthritis.

- It's antibacterial and antifungal.

- It decreases fevers.

- It aids with nausea, including the nausea of pregnancy and nausea and vomiting of chemotherapy.

- It reduces the risk of heart and cardiovascular disease by increasing circulation and preventing the clotting of blood.

- It may be used as a prophylactic for migraine headaches.

Here are some basic facts you should know about taking ginger:

- Checking for quality: Fresh is always best, but you can use dried ginger or encapsulated ginger extracts.

- Dosing: 1 to 2 grams of fresh or dried ginger a day can help with pain, aches, and inflammation. Drink 1 to 3 cups of ginger tea for aches and pains or add a 1/4-inch piece of peeled, diced ginger to your stir-fry.

    Capsules containing at least 170 milligrams of ginger root extract, taken three times a day, are helpful with arthritis.

- Caution/contraindications: Ginger may interact with blood thinners like warfarin (Coumadin), so consult your physician before adding it to your diet in large amounts. People with gallstones or those who have experienced a peptic ulcer should take caution in taking ginger, as should anyone taking antacids.

Turmeric/Curcumin

Turmeric comes from the root of the Indian Curcuma longa plant and is the main ingredient in curry. It contains an extract called curcumin that researchers have studied extensively for its multiple anti-inflammatory benefits. Curcumin lends the spice its bright orange color.

Curcumin works in much the same way as ibuprofen but without the gastrointestinal side effects. That is, it inhibits the inflammatory cascade (the competition of different cells for the same enzyme) in the body mediated by cyclooxygenase-2 (COX-2), prostaglandins, and leukotrienes. Curcumin also works as an antioxidant and stimulates the immune system.

Here are some of the anti-inflammatory benefits of curcumin:

- It helps relieve indigestion by increasing digestive enzymes.

- It has hepatoprotective effects, which protect against liver damage.

- It helps with cognitive function and may decrease the risk of dementia and Alzheimer's disease.

- It reduces the pain and inflammation symptoms of rheumatoid arthritis.

- It works as a cancer preventative by inhibiting tumor promotion, inhibiting the growth of cancer cells, and reducing their blood supply.

- It may help with circulation by preventing the platelets from clumping together.

Here are some basic facts you should know about taking curcumin:

- Checking for quality: The price of a curcumin extract may reflect its quality and standardization. The better-quality companies ensure that they have a good quality of turmeric to start and have the right amount of curcumin in each bottle, so quality extracts cost a bit more.

- Dosing: For anti-inflammatory benefit, you may need to take 500 milligrams up to three times a day. Turmeric and curcumin seem to be better absorbed with food.

- Caution/contraindications: Curcumin should not be taken by people with gallstones or obstructed bile ducts without first consulting a physician. It can increase the risk of severe bleeding, so people with bleeding disorders shouldn't take it or those who are taking blood-thinning medication.

NAC (N-acetyl cysteine)

N-acetyl cysteine (NAC) is a derivative of amino acids, the building blocks of protein. NAC reduces free-radical damage and stops inflammation by acting as an antioxidant.

Here are some of the anti-inflammatory benefits of NAC:

- It protects against drug toxicity and aspirin poisoning.

- It promotes liver detoxification.

- It helps lower the risk of cardiovascular disease by decreasing homocysteine.

- It prevents bronchitis and improves the condition of people with chronic obstructive pulmonary disease (COPD).

- It's cancer-protective.

- It increases circulation by inhibiting platelet aggregation.

- It helps protect the immune system in HIV disease.

- It helps relieve compulsive psychiatric disorders.

Here are some basic facts you should know about taking NAC:

- Checking for quality: Make sure you get your supplements from a reputable source or a doctor who specializes in nutritional supplements.

- Dosing: A general safe dose is 600 milligrams once or twice a day. Always consult your physician before starting any new herbs or supplements.

- Caution/contraindications: NAC is generally safe, although people taking blood pressure medications, diabetes medications, and anticoagulants should avoid NAC due to some gastrointestinal side effects. Pregnant women should also avoid taking NAC.

<u>Bromelain</u>

Bromelain, an enzyme derived from pineapple, decreases the inflammatory response of the immune system and works as an antioxidant to increase reactive oxygen species (ROS) that clean up the mess of inflammation.

Bromelain also helps with circulation by inhibiting platelet aggregation, and it works against cancer by disrupting the growth of cancer cells. A study in osteoarthritis of the knee showed that a combination of bromelain with other antioxidants at 50 milligrams three times a day worked as well as the medication diclofenac (Voltaren) in reducing pain and improving function.

Here are some other anti-inflammatory benefits of bromelain:

- It aids digestion.

- It helps with healing after surgery and trauma.

- It helps alleviate allergy symptoms.

- It eases aches and pains by acting as a smooth muscle relaxant, and it reduces muscle soreness after workouts.

- It has cardiovascular and circulatory applications, including the inhibition of thrombus formation and platelet aggregation.

- It helps reduce the inflammatory symptoms of inflammatory bowel diseases such as ulcerative colitis.

Here are some basic facts you should know about taking bromelain:

- Checking for quality: Make sure you get your supplements from a reputable source or a doctor who specializes in nutritional supplements.

- Dosing: 200 to 1,000 milligrams a day is generally used for arthritis and pain. It should be taken in divided doses on an empty stomach.

- Caution/contraindications: Because bromelain has anti-platelet aggregation activity, you should use it with caution alongside other medications that work the same way, such as warfarin (Coumadin) and other blood thinners. Those with allergies to pineapple should avoid this supplement.

Boswellia

Boswellia, the tree resin from the Boswellia serrata plant, is also called Indian frankincense. It contains boswellic acid, an alpha, and beta boswellic acid, which researchers found to have anti-inflammatory properties in laboratory research. The anti-inflammatory properties of the boswellic acids come from their ability to prevent the formation of chemical signals in the body for inflammation. Namely, 5 lipoxygenase, leukotrienes, and leukocyte elastase.

Boswellia is an arthritis pain reliever in that it decreases the breakdown of cartilage and helps keep the joints lubricated. For autoimmune disease, Boswellia appears to inhibit the chemical signals of autoimmune disease and reduce the formation of antibodies, the body's attack cells.

Among Boswellia's benefits are the following:

- It decreases inflammation in osteoarthritis, rheumatoid arthritis, tendonitis, bursitis, and general aches and pains.

- It's used to reduce inflammation in inflammatory bowel diseases such as ulcerative colitis and Crohn's disease.

- It may help decrease inflammation in asthma and allergies.

- It has antibacterial and antiviral properties.

- It has been shown to prevent cancer cell growth and help with programmed cancer cell death in colon cancer.

- It protects against certain autoimmune diseases and their symptoms.

Here are some basic facts you should know about taking Boswellia:

- Checking for quality: Make sure you get your supplements from a reputable source or a doctor who specializes in nutritional supplements.

- Dosing: 300 milligrams, three times a day, is generally used for arthritis and inflammatory disorders.

- Caution/contraindications: Boswellia is generally safe.

Vitamin D

Vitamin D is probably one of the most effortless nutrients to obtain, yet it is one in which the majority of people have deficiencies. Vitamin D is a fat-soluble vitamin that is stimulated in the skin by exposure to the sun and is found in small amounts in some foods. A laboratory test called 25-hydroxy vitamin D shows that most people are vitamin D deficient unless they spend time outside in full sun every day.

The following are among vitamin D's many anti-inflammatory benefits:

- It boosts the immune system.

- It prevents rickets, a disorder causing bones to become weak and deformed.

- It protects against muscle aches and pains.

- It prevents osteoporosis and osteopenia and reduces the risk of bone fracture.

- It lowers the risk of autoimmune disorders such as rheumatoid arthritis and MS, and it improves symptoms in people with such disorders.

- It helps with blood sugar regulation, and it may prevent Type 1 diabetes.

- It protects against heart and cardiovascular disease. Researchers think vitamin D does this by affecting inflammatory mediators such as tumor necrosis factor-alpha (TNF-alpha) and interleukin.

- It decreases the risk of cancer, specifically breast, prostate, and colon cancers.

Here are some basic facts you should know about vitamin D:

- Checking for quality: Make sure to use vitamin D3 rather than vitamin D2.

- Dosing: In general, most adults need 400 to 1,000 IU (international units) of vitamin D daily. However, people with autoimmune disease and who are very deficient in the vitamin may need more to achieve optimal blood levels. We list some dietary sources of vitamin D3 in Table 22-1.

Full-body sun exposure for about 12 minutes, during the sunniest part of the day (midday), produces approximately 10,000 units of vitamin D. If you're unable to get this exposure, just expose the hands, face, arms, and legs to sunlight two to three times a week. Do that for about a quarter of the time it would take you, to get a mild sunburn. That will cause the skin to produce minimal requirements of vitamin D. So, if you usually start to turn pink after 20 minutes in the sun, try for 5 minutes of sun exposure two to three times a week; that could be as easy as walking to the end of your street and back. It's important to mention, however, that a variety of factors — clothing, sunscreen, dark skin pigmentation, and air pollution, among others — can limit the sun's strength, and, therefore, the amount of vitamin D the body is stimulated to produce.

- Caution/contraindications: Toxicity due to too much vitamin D is rare; in fact, the only studies that showed toxicity used 100,000 IU or more given intravenously. You'd need 25-hydroxyvitamin D blood levels of 150 ng/mL or more to get toxicity from vitamin D.

Caution is advised with vitamin D in people with liver disease, people with high blood calcium levels, and people with granulomatous disorders such as sarcoidosis and tuberculosis (TB).

Vitamin C

Vitamin C, also known as ascorbic acid, is a water-soluble vitamin that decreases inflammation by acting as a potent antioxidant. Vitamin C also reduces C-reactive protein, the protein that gets elevated when your body is inflamed.

You can find high amounts of vitamin C in vegetables and fruits, including broccoli, papaya, bell peppers, oranges, cantaloupe, kiwi, cauliflower, Brussels sprouts, and strawberries. Overcooking and prolonged storage decrease the vitamin C content in food, so eat these fruits and vegetables raw or slightly cooked.

Among the anti-inflammatory benefits of vitamin C are the following:

- It's an antioxidant.

- It stimulates the immune system and prevents infections.

- It helps decrease allergy symptoms.

- It prevents gout by reducing uric acid levels.

- It helps people with cardiovascular disease by preventing free radical damage.

- It helps maintain connective tissue integrity to prevent wrinkles.

- It protects the skin against sun damage.

- It can be used adjunctively in cancer care or to help with cancer prevention (although consultation with an oncologist is necessary and appropriate).

- It prevents scurvy, a disease caused by a deficiency in vitamin C that includes the swelling and bleeding of the gums and the opening of previously healed wounds.

- It aids in wound healing.

- It may help in increasing HDL (good) cholesterol.

Here are some basic facts you should know about increasing your intake of vitamin C:

- Checking for quality: Vitamin C can be made synthetically in a lab or derived from food sources, such as rose hips. Food-derived sources may be better absorbed than synthetic sources because the body can't absorb more than 1 gram at a time — the rest is lost through urine.

- Dosing: You need at least 100 milligrams a day to prevent scurvy and 1 to 3 grams a day for optimal function in preventing oxidative damage due to free radicals and increasing immune support. Start with 100 milligrams a day and slowly increase to 1 to 3 grams. The upper limit of vitamin C is determined by bowel tolerance (too much vitamin C will lead to loose stools). If you hit that upper limit, begin scaling back your daily amount of vitamin C.

- Caution/contraindications: Too much vitamin C causes diarrhea and stomach upset. It's safe in doses up to the point where it causes loose stools, called bowel tolerance. For adults, the recommended daily maximum of vitamin C is 2,000 milligrams.

Papain

Papain, an enzyme derived from the fruit of the papaya plant, helps reduce inflammation by breaking down harmful substances in the body and releasing substances such as reactive oxygen species (ROS) and cytokines that reduce inflammation and have an antioxidant function.

Here are some of the papain's anti-inflammatory benefits:

- It's a digestive aid/enzyme.
- It's used to help reduce inflammation and improve healing after surgery and trauma.
- It can help prevent post-operative adhesions.
- It can help reduce inflammation of the throat and may reduce symptoms of tonsillitis.
- It aids in wound healing.

- It may reduce pain and inflammation in rheumatic disease.

Here are some basic facts you should know about taking papain:

- Checking for quality: Make sure you get your supplements from a reputable source or a doctor who specializes in nutritional supplements.

- Dosing: 1,500 milligrams a day is the dose used to treat inflammation and swelling after surgery or trauma. Take it on an empty stomach for best results.

- Caution/contraindications: Some people may be allergic to papaya and papain. People with GERD and ulcers, as well as those taking immuno-suppression therapy and radiation therapy, should be especially cautious when eating papain.

Coenzyme Q10

Coenzyme Q10 is a vitamin-like substance that provides energy to all the cells of your body. It's an antioxidant, and it helps stabilize the cell membranes. You need coenzyme Q10 to complete many of your metabolic functions. For example, the mitochondria in your cells use it to make adenosine triphosphate (ATP), your cells' primary energy source.

Among the anti-inflammatory benefits of coenzyme Q10 are the following:

- It provides energy for all the cells of your body.

- It protects the heart and body against free-radical damage.

- It reduces the risk of heart disease and helps normalize blood pressure.

- It protects the body against muscle damage due to statin (cholesterol-lowering) drugs, such as Lipitor. Statins inhibit the enzyme needed to make cholesterol and coenzyme Q10.

- It may protect the brain against damage and aids in treating Parkinson's disease.

- It helps reduce the occurrence of migraine headaches.

- It has benefits in cancer protection.

- It helps protect the gums against gingivitis.

Here are some basic facts you should know about taking coenzyme Q10:

- Checking for quality: Coenzyme Q10 needs to be in an emulsified (fat-soluble) form in order to be absorbed. Some people who have difficulty absorbing coenzyme Q10 may do better with its derivative, called ubiquinol.

- Dosing: Generally, 60 to 100 milligrams a day provides proper antioxidant protection.

- Caution/contraindications: Coenzyme Q10 looks like the blood-thinning vitamin, vitamin K, so that coenzyme Q10 may interact with other blood thinners. Have your physician monitor your blood if you're on a blood thinner such as warfarin (Coumadin).

INFLAMMATION AND ANTI-AGING

Inflammation is, in part, a well-functioning immune system that stimulates a complex series of chemical and cellular activities performed by the body in response to (1) injury or (2) abnormal stimulation caused by a physical, chemical, or biological agent. We have all heard of inflammation, felt its uncomfortable side, and dealt with it in our usual ways. But many of us do not know that there is a direct link between inflammation and aging. We are not aware that free radicals within our body are the culprit of inflammation, and factors in our everyday life trigger these free radicals that can disrupt cell function. This article will help explain that daily inflammation sustained over one's lifetime is the hidden cause of aging and disease. It will examine the causes of inflammation and will offer opportunities, through diet and supplementation, to control these abnormal cellular activities, providing a healthy age management lifestyle.

Aging is inevitable, but how one ages is a choice. Some people seem to age well, looking younger than their actual birth date; others appear to be a decade older than their chronological age. Our genetic makeup helps determine how we age, but there are other factors just as important. Medical intervention has helped extend lifespan. While the average lifespan in 1900 was approximately 46 to 48 years, today, individuals can expect to live well into their eighties. But how one lives these years, and how well chronic illness is kept at bay, is highly dependent on anti-aging factors.

The "free radical theory of aging" examines the factors that impact our genes and provides a foundation for how we age. In simple terms, the theory explains how mutations occur and how we can prevent and overcome aging problems that result from injury, infection, or DNA damage. The message is that free radicals within the body are the leading cause of inflammation, resulting in disease. Control free radical damage through dietary choices and supplementation of antioxidants, and you control damage to DNA.

Denham Harman, a medical physics researcher at the University of California, Berkeley, conceived the "free radical theory of aging" in 1956. Free radicals are highly charged atoms that are missing one electron, making them unstable. They enter our body through sunlight, poor diet, use of alcohol, tobacco, airborne chemicals, even stress, and steal an electron in order to gain chemical stability. Favorite targets are fatty acids; cell membranes that are rich in phospholipids; DNA, and proteins. When targeted orderly cellular processes are replaced by the utter chaos of electron swapping that eventually disrupts cell function. Free radicals are considered the primary culprits in aging because they produce random radical change and deviation from a well-ordered healthy cellular metabolism. As a consequence, free radicals produce inflammation, and daily inflammation sustained over a lifetime is the cause of aging and disease. Certain signs of inflammation include swelling, heat, pain in joints, and redness. As we age, our defenses decline, and our tissues accumulate the end products of oxidative damage. We notice our skin is wrinkling, or perhaps we are accumulating "age spots." On the inside of our body, oxidative stress damages key molecules essential to our DNA, causing cancer, diabetes, heart disease, poor circulation, and other age-associated diseases.

DNA is particularly sensitive to oxidative stress. As electrons are stolen, they leave "pits" in the individual strands of DNA. Free radicals cause strands of DNA to break and wear away. The resulting nicks and strand breaks affect both functioning cells and stem cells. Stem cell damage is extremely devastating since these cells are precursors for thousands of different kinds of cells found in the body. Since the significant role of stem cells is the reproduction, damaged stem cells affect future generations of all functioning cells. Cancer is one disease that depends on DNA damage. A familiar example of this is the many forms of skin cancer.

Inflammation is a dominant defensive mechanism of the body's immune system. Once a foreign body is detected, the immune system responds with inflammation, characterized by redness, swelling, and pain at the site of infection. The same things that trigger free radicals cause inflammation. Sunlight, smog, airborne chemicals, poor diet, alcohol, drugs, smoking, and stress are all causes of inflammation. Acute inflammation occurs in response to an injury or infection. Usually, within a 24 to 48-hour period, this phase resolves itself, and the recovery process begins. Cellular garbage is removed from the site of injury, and healthy replacement tissue grows. As we age, our antioxidant defenses decline, and the oxidative damage causes chronic inflammatory conditions. This type of inflammation is more prolonged. Free radicals, severe stress, and environmental agents do not respond to immune attack. There is no recovery process, and severe pain and tissue damage occur. Overcoming these conditions and reversing aging depends on efficient DNA repair. Our question is, how can we help nature along a repair process for DNA and reverse aging? One way is through diet and supplementation. How you lead your life is another way. Both approaches are choices.

Appropriate diet, supplementation, and lifestyle choices are essential to preventing inflammation, neutralizing free radicals, and promoting healthy age management. Among our choices, there are acid and alkaline based foods. Diet should consist of 80% alkaline foods and 20% acidic foods. A rainbow selection of six servings of fruits and vegetables, organic whenever possible, can assure this all-important acid/alkaline balance, reducing inflammation through providing the body with a multitude of antioxidants. Carrots, pumpkin, peppers, tomatoes, mangos, and papaya are all orange and "red coded" and protect our genes. Asparagus, broccoli, Pak choy, onions, and mustard greens are 'green coded' and help improve cellular nutrients and detoxify our body. Blackberries, cherries, beets are purple and blue and reduce inflammation. Barley, mushrooms, tofu, and wild rice are tan and reduce insulin resistance and balance hormones. Herbs and spices, such as garlic, turmeric, cinnamon, curry, ginger, and cayenne help to neutralize free radicals.

Generally, meats, grains, nuts, and sugar are acidic and promote unhealthy free radicals. Meats should be free-range, meaning that they are free of hormones and antibiotics. One should have a diet of farm-raised salmon, tilapia, flounder, and sardines and avoid swordfish, which is known to be high in mercury. Barley, quinoa, brown rice, and wild rice are excellent choices of grains. Nuts and seeds are important to a well-rounded diet. Dark leafy greens, legumes, and red, yellow, orange, and green vegetables must be consumed with each meal to balance the necessary acidic foods which offer us the much-needed protein, vitamins, and minerals our body needs. We can further reduce inflammation with high levels of alkaline water intake, green tea, and avoiding sugar, vinegar, salt, and corn syrup. In a nutshell, emphasize lean organic protein, and combine vegetable sources, eat selectively, avoid sugary sweets, nitrates, nitrites, smoked meats, and trans-fats, watch portion sizes, do not eat on the run, and chew your food. You should have five servings of fruits and vegetables, preferably green and orange-red color selection. Drink plenty of liquids between meals; no soda, eat meals at regular times; do not eat late, and avoid processed foods. Reduce dairy consumption. We are the only species that consumes another species' milk!

Many anti-inflammatory supplements are antioxidants and help our body control free radical damage. High-quality multivitamin/mineral complex is essential to a healthy lifestyle. Folic acids, B vitamins, vitamins D, C, A, E, Boswellia, Glucosamine-Chondroitin, curcumin, molecularly distilled Omega 3 and 6 from cold-water fish Tri-Methylglycine, CoQ Enzyme 10, R-Lipoic Acid, and Resveratrol are all supplements that will slow down disease progression and reduce inflammation. Vitamins A, C, and E lower the risk of heart disease. They reduce inflammation and protect against induced oxidative damage. Those with diabetes can see improvement in "insulin action." Green tea protects against estrogenic breast cancer. Vitamin D3 prevents colon cancer, and aged garlic prevents damage to DNA and also reduces inflammation. Generally, by increasing detoxification, we rid our bodies of free radicals.

The use of the enzyme CoQ10 has significant results in curbing aging. This supplement prevents oxidative damage to the brain, enhances speedy recovery and cardiac function from heart attacks, and prevents thyroid disorders. Alpha-Lipoic acid improves carbohydrate metabolism, improves brain energy and muscular-skeletal performance, and "soaks" up free radicals within the body.

Diet, supplementation, and knowledge are the key ingredients to age management. But lifestyle changes complete the entire picture in promoting lifespan. Research shows that stress initiates profound changes in cellular structure that lead to aging diseases, particularly those involving inflammation and immune function. Work towards eliminating stress, and you prolong your lifespan. Daily exercise, prayer, and meditation are also positive forces to incorporate into one's life. Learn to be mindful, develop a relationship with your God, and think "holistically." Reduce alcohol consumption, aid your digestive process with probiotics, improve proper alimentation, and decrease acidic foods. There is no magic bullet, but a desire for wellness becomes a lifestyle that comes bearing extraordinary gifts for a life of feeling good and looking good. True beauty comes from within. There are no shortcuts!

ANTI-INFLAMMATORY FOODS

Almost everyone these days seems to have some understanding of the basic food pyramid: fruits, vegetables, grains, dairy, and meat. Making sure you get the proper number of servings of each group has been a nutritional mainstay in the United States since the early 1990s, and it's spilled over to other countries as well.

For people fighting inflammation, not only can following the basic food guidelines be inadequate, but it can also aid inflammation, contributing to problems such as diabetes, heart disease, and even certain cancers. Figuring out which foods help in the battle against inflammation and knowing how much of each food you need is a great start to changing to an anti-inflammatory lifestyle. That can not only improve how you feel now, but it can also help you make great strides in overall health.

This chapter guides you through the basic food pyramid — and the USDA's new plate image — and the best adjustments you can make to change your menu from one that aids in inflammation to one that fights it.

An anti-inflammatory diet is not designed to help you lose weight (although weight loss is a good possibility because inflammation influences your weight), nor is this diet something that you should consider temporary. Committing to an anti-inflammatory diet is telling yourself that you want to do what you can to get and stay healthy.

Following Recommendations for Good and Bad Food Categories

The food recommendations for an anti-inflammation diet are geared toward keeping your body healthy. These recommendations steer you toward (or away from) both specific foods and general types of foods, so you can design your menu based on what you know.

Here are some good-food categories to keep in mind when changing to an anti-inflammatory diet:

- Omega-3 fatty acids: You can find these fats, which can help reduce inflammation, in cold-water oily fish, walnuts, flaxseeds, and olive oil. None of those sound appealing? Omega-3 fatty acids are available in supplement form as well.

- Protein: Protein helps build healthy tissues and keeps inflammation at bay. That is where your lean poultry, fish, nuts, and legumes fit in. Protein sources that are high in fiber and nutrients, like legumes, help to decrease inflammation by balancing blood sugar, providing the building blocks to build muscle, and giving you long-term energy.

- Fiber: Here's where your fruits and vegetables, as well as whole grains, come into play. All these foods are rich in fiber, which helps your body fight inflammation. Good news for pasta-lovers is that brown rice pasta makes the list of good-for-you fibers.

- Water: Although your body gets some water in the form of fruits and vegetables, drinking plenty of water every day is still a great idea. Don't like plain water? Use it to make herbal teas or find fruit juices that are 100 percent juice and dilute them with water to keep the sugar concentrations down.

Here are some bad-food categories to avoid when changing to an anti-inflammatory diet:

- Sugars: Researchers have found that sugar increases the risk of obesity, inflammation, and diabetes. Look instead for natural sweeteners, such as honey, agave nectar, pure maple syrup, brown rice syrup, or stevia. For information on sugars and sweeteners, turn to Chapter 8.

- Omega-6 fatty acids: Many of the most common cooking oils are high in omega-6 fatty acids, and diets high in these fats are inflammatory and can lead to increased risks of cancer and heart disease. Reach for the extra-virgin olive oil and the other oils.

- Trans fats: Trans fats, which for a long time appeared in most fast foods, fried foods, and commercial baked goods, do the opposite of what they should: They lower the good cholesterol and raise the bad cholesterol, increasing the risks of obesity and insulin resistance. Many food producers have reformulated recipes, so trans fats aren't as plentiful, but these bad fats are still out there, so be sure to read food labels carefully.

- Dairy products: More than half of the U.S. population has some degree of lactose intolerance and sensitivity to all or some dairy products. This sensitivity can lead to poor digestion, diarrhea, constipation, and stomach distress.

- Meats: Particularly avoid meats from feedlot-fed animals, red meats, and processed meats, which you find in most supermarkets and restaurants. These meats are high in omega-6 fatty acids, and processed meats have been smoked, cured, or otherwise treated with chemicals. Smoking meats creates nitrosamines, which have been linked to intestinal and breast cancer. Curing isn't that bad unless it involves using preservatives, and in many cases soaking in a salt brine is used as well.

- Refined or enriched grains: Most of the grains found on store shelves or used in baked goods have been stripped of the plant's bulk, which contains the nutritional properties. Refined grains are more powdery and less coarse, and they can speed up the development of cancer and heart disease.

Adapting General Food Recommendations for Your Needs

The food pyramid Americans have come to know — which the United States Department of Agriculture (USDA) introduced in 1992 and revised in 2005 — has long been a symbol of healthy eating and maintaining balance. It offered guidelines for people to follow a balanced menu incorporating foods from each of five groups — fruits, vegetables, grains, meat, and milk — with limited amounts of fats, oils, and sweets.

The USDA acknowledged the pyramid's shortcomings and, in June 2011, did away with the pyramid, replacing it with a simplified symbol of a divided plate. The new plate is divided into portions indicating areas for fruits, vegetables, grains, protein (replacing the meat group), and dairy. Fruits and vegetables take up half of the plate, and grains and protein share the other half. Dairy is located where a glass would be in a place setting.

What the food guidelines still don't do is address the individual needs of people fighting inflammation or people trying to stave off diabetes or cancer or heart ailments. How can whole grains and pasta hurt you if you're fighting inflammation? Is having red meat every day a good idea? Are there dangers in certain fruits and vegetables?

In this section, we transform the traditional food pyramid, identifying which foods don't fit with an anti-inflammatory diet, which foods to add, and how to make a new anti-inflammatory pyramid that works for you. We also discuss the latest USDA recommendations and the agency's new food plate for nutrition, identifying how it differs from the iconic food pyramid and why we stick with the pyramid to present anti-inflammatory recommendations.

Herbs and spices: Going beyond the five food groups

The USDA's food pyramid and plate stress the importance of getting something from each of the five food groups. They even recommend how much of each you should eat. But the guidelines stop with these food categories. Other foods, spices, and extras should be a part of your diet as you're fighting inflammation or inflammation-related issues.

A lot of herbs and spices offer many benefits because they contain phytochemicals (the compounds produced by plants), bioflavonoids (the anti-oxidants found in fruits and vegetables), omega-3 fatty acids, and other anti-inflammatory nutrients that enhance the natural foods from the food pyramid.

Here are some of the top anti-inflammatory herbs and spices and what they can do:

- Cayenne pepper: Works to kill some cancer cells and clean out the arteries.

- Cumin: Helps flush toxins from the body and prevents and fights cancers.

- Garlic: Is anti-inflammatory because of its high sulfur content and has antiviral and antibacterial properties as well.

- Ginger: It also helps with inflammations causing joint pain. (It's an excellent natural way to beat headaches, too!)

- Turmeric: Helps relieve arthritis, tendonitis, and even some autoimmune disorders.

Other herbs and spices that aid in the fight against inflammation are black pepper, cinnamon, rosemary, basil, cardamom, chives, cilantro, cloves, and parsley.

When adding herbs and spices to a favorite food, stick to the serving size of about 1/2 to 1 teaspoon to get the optimum effect. When using fresh herbs, you can be a bit more generous, using roughly twice as much fresh than you would use dried. With fresh ginger, use at least a 1-inch piece to get valuable medicinal benefits. Both dried and fresh herbs and spices have great anti-inflammatory benefits.

Creating the anti-inflammatory food pyramid

The traditional food pyramid offers guidelines for the number of servings a "normal" person should have in terms of fruits, vegetables, milk, meats and beans, and grains. The new plate identifies the food groups — replacing meats with proteins — but doesn't define how much of each you should have. The new plate even provides altered menus for those with special needs, such as pregnant and breastfeeding women, preschoolers, and people pursuing weight loss.

What the plate doesn't do, however, is take into account people whose diets are limited by sensitivities, allergies, or chronic inflammation. Not everyone can tolerate dairy products or grains, and people who are fighting inflammation won't be reaching for red meats or certain vegetables and fruits.

Some foods are more likely than others to be associated with sensitivities, creating even more problems for the body. For example, wheat and dairy can create problems even for people not suffering from celiac disease or lactose intolerance, and corn, eggs, and citrus fruits can cause heightened sensitivities as well. Additionally, eating the same thing too many times in a short time frame, such as a week, can lead to sensitization to the food, and the body may start attacking what is usually known as "good" food, thinking it's something foreign.

We've taken the traditional food pyramid and altered it to address just those issues, specifying the inclusion of gluten-free grains, providing alternatives to dairy, and identifying meats and proteins other than red meats.

Getting the full benefits of an anti-inflammatory diet means knowing just how much is enough and then following through. Striking the right nutritional balance is just as important as knowing which foods to eat. For the most part, if you play by the anti-inflammatory rules at least 90 percent of the time, you'll still feel optimum benefits of fighting inflammation.

How Foods Stack Up Based on Inflammation Factors

Researchers at the University of South Carolina and the University of Massachusetts created an inflammation index in 2009 in an effort to see just how inflammatory peoples' diets are. After examining nearly 60 years' worth of reports, studies, and articles on foods and how their compounds can affect the body, researchers scored foods according to whether they were anti-inflammatory or inflammatory. That means, whether they helped to prevent or alleviate inflammation or whether they were part of the problem.

Researchers then gave each food an inflammation factor (IF) rating based on whether it was anti-inflammatory. Foods with positive IF Ratings are considered anti-inflammatory, and foods with negative ratings contribute to the development of inflammation.

The formula used to determine each food's IF rating takes into consideration more than 20 factors, including the type and amount of fat in each food, the levels of vitamins and other nutrients, and any anti-inflammatory compounds that may be present. Each food carries the same IF rating for everyone, but your body is going to react to each food differently.

Want to know whether that grapefruit you're eating in the morning is better than a plain bagel with cream cheese? Check out the nutritional breakdown feature on http://nutritiondata.self.com. Just enter a food item into the search box at the top of the home page and click Search to see its IF rating and other nutritional info. That grapefruit has an IF rating of 18, and the bagel and cream cheese get a –640!

Researchers also set a target daily IF value, providing the opportunity to balance anti- and inflammatory foods. The goal of the IF rating is to end the day with an IF score of at least 50. That doesn't mean you need to, or even you should avoid foods with negative IF ratings. Instead, use the rating system as a tool for balance: If you're not lactose intolerant, it's okay to have a cup of plain yogurt, even though it has an IF rating of –71. Balance that yogurt out with a small spinach salad with olive oil for lunch (one cup of raw spinach has an IF rating of 78 and a teaspoon of olive oil scores 24, for a total of 102). By the end of lunch, your net IF score is 31.

In the following sections, we identify which foods are more inflammatory than others, and which you should be adding to your diet. We list possible problems with various kinds of foods and how likely it is that you may find yourself experiencing some of these issues.

Steering clear of inflammatory foods

Although splurging occasionally is okay, certain foods are highly inflammatory and should be avoided. Such foods include high-omega-6 oils (such as those made from corn, safflower, sunflower, and cottonseed), inflammatory saturated fats from animal sources (as found in processed meats like bologna and hot dogs), and refined sugars and trans fats. Minimize or eliminate the amount of processed food and fast food you eat. Many of these foods are high in starch and sugars, as well as refined flours. For people with certain allergies or sensitivities, gluten products (wheat, barley, and rye), soy products, corn and corn products, and foods in the nightshade family (potatoes, tomatoes, and eggplant) can be highly inflammatory.

Here are some of the more common inflammatory foods to avoid and their IF ratings:

- Bread, rolls, bagels, pancakes, waffles: –4 to –51;

- Baked goods including cookies, cakes, doughnuts, and muffins: –107 to –300;

- Cereals (except old-fashioned oatmeal): –121 to –200

- Corn syrup: –63 per teaspoon to –1,100 per cup;

- Crackers, tortillas: –170;

- Fruit juices, soda: –50;

- Fried foods: –80 to –200;

- Hard cheeses, particularly nonorganic: –120;

- Ice cream and frozen yogurt: –84 to –157 (frozen yogurt is a lot worse);

- Jams and jellies: –65;

- Pasta made with white flour: –57;

- Potatoes: –88.

The easiest way to determine if a food is going to work for or against you is to simply look at the food and its label. Especially from the label, you will recognize whether a food is anti-inflammatory or inflammatory. The less "natural" a food seems to be, the higher the possibility that it's going to be inflammatory.

In the ingredients list, look for words like refined, enriched, and processed — all words that let you know something has been done to the food or the ingredients to make it as it is now. Refined sugars, for example, means the product has been stripped of everything but the chemical compound sucrose, so all the plant's nutritional elements are lost.

In some cases, using organic or natural products in place of those that are more commercially produced can improve the food's inflammation factor. Still, sometimes it's just best to do without the food altogether.

Knowing which foods are inflammatory can be as simple as keeping one rule of thumb in mind: If it doesn't look like it did originally, it's probably inflammatory. For example, whole grains, such as bulgur wheat, brown rice, and oats, all look like they do in the wild: complete with the germ and the entire grain kernel. After those grains become refined, they take on an entirely different appearance. For example, refined brown rice becomes starchy white rice.

That's not to say that you have to eat everything raw. You can change a food's appearance on your own after you have it in the kitchen: Food can be cut, crushed, steamed, and so on. Chapter 16 gives you advice on making your home cooking endeavors less inflammatory.

Hailing the anti-inflammatory foods

The good news is that there are plenty of functional foods that can help prevent or lessen inflammation. Anti-inflammatory foods are those that make you feel better and reduce your risk of inflammation and chronic disease. Whole, natural foods top the list. Processed meats and most red meats are no-no's, but lean poultry, fish, and even some red meat such as venison and bison go a long way in fighting inflammation.

Most fruits and vegetables, particularly those grown organically and eaten fresh rather than canned, pass the muster on the list of anti-inflammatory foods. They're just naturally good for you. The following sections highlight some anti-inflammatory foods and their IF ratings.

Onions

Like garlic, onions have high sulfur content. They also have antiviral and antibacterial properties. The World Health Organization (WHO) recognizes the health benefits of onions and supports their use in the treatment of atherosclerosis (hardened arteries). Onions are rich in fructooligosaccharides, which are very beneficial in colon health. One cup of diced raw onions has an IF rating of 374, and one tablespoon has a rating of 23.

Mushrooms

Mushrooms are anti-inflammatory. Most edible mushrooms are full of proteins, beneficial vitamins and minerals, and antioxidants and amino acids. They also contain polysaccharides (complex carbohydrates) that are good for the immune system. The most beneficial edible mushrooms are the Asian, maitake, oyster, and shiitake mushrooms. These mushrooms should be eaten cooked, not raw.

Mushrooms have a small negative IF rating — maitake mushrooms, for example, have an IF rating of –9 for one cup — but their other health benefits outweigh that rating.

On their own, mushrooms provide good protein with zero cholesterol and fats; some mushrooms can help to lower cholesterol levels. The beta-glucans and linoleic acid levels have anti-carcinogen benefits, helping battle breast and prostate cancer. Mushrooms are also rich in calcium, vitamin D, iron, potassium, and selenium, so they help lower blood pressure and fight anemia while helping to strengthen bones. The first statins discovered were found in medicinal molds, and the oyster mushroom naturally contains a statin.

Fermented foods

Fermented foods — those that microorganisms have partially broken down — are active fighters against inflammation because they still contain the good bacteria, yeast, or mold that many processing practices kill off. Fermented foods include cheese, miso, kimchi, yogurt, sauerkraut, vinegar, sour cream, olives, and pickles.

The IF ratings for fermented foods vary; for example, sauerkraut and vinegar are slightly anti-inflammatory, while miso and sour cream are mild to strongly inflammatory. There is no standard for this food category, but you can find the ratings for each food at http://nutritiondata.self.com.

Fermented foods are easier to digest (although fermented dairy products should be avoided if you have dairy sensitivities). They also aid in the absorption of certain nutrients and enzymes within the fermented foods.

SUPPLEMENTS TO REDUCE INFLAMMATION

In addition to refining your diet, finding supplements to boost your immune system and keep inflammation at bay can keep you feeling your best.

Pharmaceutical drugs, which are generally synthetic creations of laboratory work, are designed to prevent or treat a particular condition. Medications are typically developed to be potent and to work for the body; they, therefore, have not only strong activity but also some potentially strong side effects. Herbs and supplements, on the other hand, generally work with the body because they contain dietary ingredients — compounds that are recognized by the body based on the food you eat (vitamins, minerals, phytochemicals, and so on).

That's not to say that there's always a clear line between drugs and supplements. Herbal medicine is the oldest system of medicine. Many drugs were initially derived from plants and were later synthesized in the lab for consistency of the active constituents (chemical compounds that do what the drug is supposed to be used for).

In this chapter, we talk about over-the-counter drugs (particularly anti-inflammatory drugs such as NSAIDs), discuss some supplements you may want to consider, and give you some guidelines on choosing supplements wisely.

Exploring how anti-inflammatory drugs work

Inflammation doesn't just happen. Your body's cells send out signals to cell receptors, and how those receptors interpret what they're being told may lead to inflammation. For example, your body produces prostaglandins, chemicals that promote inflammation, soreness, and fever to get the immune system's defenses going to fight infection or illness.

Prostaglandins are produced by the cyclooxygenase (COX) enzyme, and there are two such enzymes: COX-1 and COX-2. Drugs that work to block or reduce inflammation — nonsteroidal anti-inflammatory drugs (NSAIDs) — do so by blocking the COX enzymes and reducing the prostaglandins.

The COX-1 enzyme also produces prostaglandins that support platelets and protect the stomach. Using NSAIDs also reduces these prostaglandins, which can cause ulcers and other issues.

Navigating your way through over-the-counter drugs

One type of pain reliever is acetaminophen, commonly sold as Tylenol or Panadol. In some cases, acetaminophen pain relievers also contain caffeine or decongestants and are promoted to treat a combination of symptoms, most often as cold relief or flu relief, and may treat a runny nose or chest congestion in addition to the pain. Acetaminophen relieves pain and reduces fevers but doesn't fight inflammation.

Most over-the-counter pain relievers are NSAIDs — nonsteroidal anti-inflammatory drugs. NSAIDs relieve the pain and reduce swelling of inflammation. Ibuprofen, naproxen, and ketoprofen (sold as Advil, Aleve, and Orudis, respectively) do a better job of relieving pain than acetaminophen or aspirin. Still, the other drugs have their advantages. Doctors often suggest acetaminophen for arthritis relief because it's gentler on the stomach, and aspirin does have some effect on the risks of heart attack (see the next section for details).

There are several different categories of NSAIDs, including salicylic acids, propionic acids, acetic acids, enolic acids, fenamic acids, napthylalkanones, pyran carboxylic acids, pyrroles, and COX-2 inhibitors. Talk to your doctor or physician to get an idea of which one may be right for you.

Although a variety of prescription and nonprescription anti-inflammatory medications are available, there's no real proof that one is better or stronger than any other. Differences lie instead in how individual inflammation sufferers respond to various medications and the risks for side effects. Some people may be able to take the NSAIDs like ibuprofen or naproxen without incident, and others may need something milder, and that doesn't upset their digestive systems or cause other problems.

<u>**Using aspirin for heart disease:**</u>

Take two and call me in the morning

Almost everyone's heard of the benefits of aspirin in heart patients. For people who've had cardiovascular events — a heart attack, for example — taking an aspirin a day helps reduce the risk of a recurrence.

Aspirin works by interfering in your blood's clotting capabilities. With atherosclerosis, your arteries begin to narrow because of a buildup of fatty deposits, commonly referred to as hardening of the arteries, and those fat deposits can burst. A blood clot then forms and can block the artery or can detach and move elsewhere in the circulatory system, preventing blood flow to the heart or the brain and causing a heart attack or stroke. Aspirin acts as a blood thinner, keeping the blood from clotting and possibly preventing the blockage of the artery.

According to the Mayo Clinic, aspirin therapy has different effects on men and women. In men of all ages, one aspirin a day may prevent a first and second heart attack and reduce the risk of heart disease. In women under age 65, taking one aspirin daily can prevent a first stroke and a second heart attack and help reduce the risk of heart disease. In women over age 65, aspirin therapy can do all that as well as prevent a first heart attack. That's the good news about aspirin therapy.

Daily aspirin therapy isn't for everyone. If you've never had a heart attack or stroke, taking a preventative daily aspirin could create a more significant danger than a heart attack or stroke. In 2009, about 50 million Americans were taking low-dose aspirin — 325 milligrams or less — a day to prevent heart disease. Some had had previous cardiovascular events or stroke, but many were taking the pills as a primary preventive measure. Researchers discovered, however, that daily use of aspirin for those who hadn't had a heart attack or stroke was not only unnecessary but posed certain health risks of its own. There is potential for causing a hemorrhagic stroke (which is a rupture of a blood vessel in the brain) or intestinal bleeding.

Before stopping daily aspirin therapy, discuss your options with your physician. A sudden stop in medication can trigger a heart attack or stroke.

You can use omega-3 fatty acids, found in fish or fish oil, to do some of the same things as aspirin but without all the unwanted side effects. Omega-3 fatty acids reduce pain, prevent platelet aggregation, and lower the risk of heart attacks and stroke.

Using Dietary Supplements to Fill in the Nutritional Gaps

According to the Food and Drug Administration (FDA), a dietary supplement is "a product taken by mouth that contains a 'dietary ingredient' intended to supplement the diet." A supplement may include anything that's naturally derived that is not a drug, including vitamins, minerals, herbs, amino acids, and some naturally derived hormone-like substances.

Supplements generally aren't as fast-acting as drugs, but some supplements are just as effective without the side effects. Supplements tend to be safer for long-term use. Vitamins and minerals such as calcium, magnesium, and vitamin D are used on a daily basis. People may use herbs and supplements short-term for acute issues (echinacea for colds), as a substitute for the pharmaceutical medication (red yeast rice for statins, which lower cholesterol), and short-term or long-term for medical conditions (quercetin for acute allergies).

This section covers some supplements you may want to consider.

Not all supplements are safe, and you can face problems if you don't know how to take supplements correctly. Work with a physician or herbalist who's been trained in drug, nutrient, and food interactions. We discuss choosing supplements safely later in "Choosing Dietary Supplements Wisely."

Taking vitamins as a defense against inflammation

We're sure you've heard it: Don't forget to take your vitamins! By increasing your daily intake of vitamins — either through supplements or by eating more of the foods that contain them — you can help keep inflammation at bay and curb the pain of existing inflammation.

Getting all the vitamins you need from food can be difficult, so consider taking a multivitamin (ask your doctor about the right kind and amount for you). Multivitamins have been shown to decrease the risk of hospitalizations and many diseases, thereby helping to reduce healthcare costs.

A vitamin's recommended daily dosage means the amount of the vitamin needed to prevent a deficiency, but that amount doesn't give you therapeutic nor optimal benefits. Always consult with your physician before taking high doses of vitamins and minerals because they can cause other nutrient imbalances or be potentially toxic.

Vitamins

Vitamins, particularly B6, B9 (folic acid), and B12, are high on the list of vitamins that have heart-protective properties. B6 is also prescribed to people with arthritis because at high doses, it shrinks the inflamed membranes around the arthritis-affected joints.

Food sources of B vitamins vary according to each vitamin: B1, also called thiamin, is in egg yolks, whole-grain bread, brown rice, green leafy vegetables, and legumes; B2, or riboflavin, is in eggs, milk, whole-grain products, and peas; B3, or niacin, is in meats, eggs, legumes, peanuts, fish, and potatoes; B6, or pyridoxine, is in liver, meat, brown rice, fish, butter, wheat germ, and soybeans; B9, or folic acid, is in green vegetables, liver, and whole-grain cereals; and B12 is in liver, meat, egg yolk, poultry, and milk.

Vitamin D

Vitamin D helps slow or prevent osteoporosis, high blood pressure, cancer, and several autoimmune diseases. It aids in the absorption of calcium, which helps the body maintain strong, healthy bones. The benefits of vitamin D also show up in the dentist's chair, reducing gingivitis (inflammation of the gums).

The best source of vitamin D is unfiltered sunlight, which triggers your skin to make its vitamin D. Good dietary sources of vitamin D include cold-water oily fish such as sardines, herring, and wild salmon.

Vitamin E

Vitamin E has powerful anti-inflammatory properties. It's been clinically proven to help reduce the risk of heart disease, Alzheimer's, arthritis, and hay fever.

The recommended daily dosage of vitamin E is about 30 International Units (IU), or about 20 milligrams. A general daily dose of 400 IU mixed tocopherols may help reducing oxidation.

Alpha-tocopherol, one of the forms of vitamin E, and synthetic forms of vitamin E increase the risk of heart disease when you take them in high amounts. Be sure to look for "mixed tocopherols," and nonsynthetic vitamin E. Mixed tocopherols are a mixture of the natural forms of vitamin E found in food, such as almonds.

Too much vitamin E has been linked to increased instances of bleeding. Although everyone should check with his or her medical practitioner before starting any kind of supplement or vitamin program, people who take blood-thinning medication or who have vitamin K deficiency should take particular caution.

Finding the benefits of fish oil tablets

Fish oil can be a healthy lifestyle addition. Fish oil is filled with the essential omega-3 fatty acids and provides health benefits for a variety of issues, from heart disease and cancer to eye disorders and skin disease. Here are a few of the area's omega-3s affect:

- Brain function: The presence of omega-3 fatty acids in fish oils has a mood-stabilizing effect, calming anxiety and depression, and treating bipolar disorder. These good fats are especially important in helping the brain's cells, or neurons, to signal each other effectively, so omega-3s also help control Alzheimer's disease. DHA also plays a role in serotonin and dopamine metabolism, having a positive effect on mood.

- Obesity and heart health: Omega-3s can help alleviate the problems associated with obesity, including heart disease and diabetes. The American Heart Association touts fish oil as playing a vital role in reducing the risk of heart disease by lowering the LDL (bad) cholesterol and raising the HDL (good) cholesterol and preventing triglycerides from getting out of control. Fish oils prevent platelet aggregation (they act as blood thinners) and help with heart arrhythmias.

- Gastrointestinal disorders: Fish oil is anti-inflammatory and has proven effective in the treatment and prevention of digestive disorders like Crohn's disease, ulcerative colitis, and irritable bowel disorders (IBD).

- Immune system: Research suggests that making fish oil a regular part of your diet can boost your immune system and help reduce the risk of inflammation in rheumatoid arthritis and autoimmune diseases.

The best natural sources of fish oil are, not surprisingly, fish. The problem with fresh fish, however, is that thanks to pollutants such as mercury, arsenic, lead, PCBs (polychlorinated biphenyls), and other substances in the waters, the oils found in fish are often contaminated.

Pharmaceutical grade fish oils are a supplement that most physicians, holistic or otherwise, can agree on as being a vital supplement for reducing the risk of cardiovascular disease and inflammation. Fish oil tablets, particularly those of good quality, provide a more than adequate substitute for the real thing, allowing your body to get the full benefits of the essential omega-3 fatty acids. To get a good quality fish oil, choose a brand that's tested for heavy metals, that's shelf-stable, and that isn't synthetic.

Fish oils do not have the toxic side effects on the gastrointestinal system and liver that the pharmaceutical drugs like aspirin have. They have more of a generalized anti-inflammatory benefit, rather than a targeted specific pathway. Addressing just a specific pathway increases the potential for side effects.

Getting a boost from mighty magnesium

You'd be hard-pressed to find a system in your body that doesn't depend on magnesium. It plays a vital role in the health of your cardiovascular, digestive, muscular, skeletal, and nervous systems, as well as your brain, kidneys, and liver. Magnesium helps blood pressure stay low, serves as a bone strengthener, and can help alleviate problems associated with the metabolic disorder — obesity, diabetes, and high cholesterol levels. More than 300 enzymes in the body need magnesium to ensure they're doing their jobs properly.

Studies show that a deficiency in magnesium can lead to elevated C-reactive protein (CRP) levels, which can, in turn, lead to heart disease and other inflammatory diseases (see Chapter 3 for details). That said, the majority of Americans — a whopping 68 percent — don't even come close to getting the recommended daily allowance (RDA) of magnesium. Some of the signs of magnesium deficiency are muscle weakness, heart arrhythmia, headaches, elevated blood pressure, depression, nausea, vomiting, and lack of appetite.

Some of the best dietary sources for magnesium are spinach, Swiss chard, mustard greens, broccoli, and summer squash. It's also available in a supplement form, both in chelated and nonchelated (connected with another molecule or not connected) forms. There are many forms of magnesium, but magnesium citrate is well absorbed and doesn't create loose stools as may occur with other forms.

An overabundance of magnesium can lead to magnesium toxicity, symptoms of which include diarrhea, drowsiness, and weakness. Be sure to check with a healthcare provider before starting on any supplemental form. The safest way to get a boost in magnesium is through your diet.

Taking herbal supplements and spices

Many herbs and spices don't just add a little zing to the flavor of your food; they also provide a flurry of anti-inflammatory benefits, from putting an end to migraines to reducing your risk of certain cancers and heart disease. Knowing what to use and how to use herbs and spices is one big step in the fight against inflammation (see Chapter 22 for details on the ten most powerful natural supplements).

Most herbs and spices are available in food form, as well as in capsules and tincture. Food form is the safest and easiest to find.

Here's a list of some of the most common herbs and spices with anti-inflammatory benefits:

- **Ginger:** Ginger calms a weak stomach and is a safe end to vomiting during pregnancy, but its healthful benefits go much further. Ginger contains very powerful anti-inflammatory compounds called gingerols that help relieve the pain of arthritis and osteoarthritis. Those same gingerols provide protection against colorectal cancer and ovarian cancer.

- **Turmeric:** This spice was first used as a dye in India more than 2,500 years ago, but it's now a common ingredient in many Indian dishes. Turmeric is one of the most potent natural spices available, with anti-cancer properties that work against pancreatic, colon, and breast cancer as well as melanoma and leukemia. Turmeric helps fight Alzheimer's disease and multiple sclerosis, and it works as a natural painkiller and antibacterial agent when used as a disinfectant for cuts and burns. (You can find more information about turmeric in Chapter 22.)

- **Aloe vera:** Aloe vera has long been known for its soothing properties in healing external cuts and sunburns, but it has some pretty powerful anti-inflammatory benefits when ingested as well. Aloe vera can cool inflammation in the digestive tract, as with peptic ulcers, and has been used to defeat problems with the liver in some countries, such as China. Take caution, however: Aloe vera can cause hypoglycemia and have a laxative effect. It counteracts with some medications, so consult with a health care provider before taking aloe vera.

- **Licorice:** Licorice has healing qualities for colds and coughs, and it also works against chronic hepatitis. People with elevated blood pressure should take caution, however; too much licorice may increase blood pressure in some people when used long term. For this reason, holistic practitioners frequently use a form of licorice root that's had glycyrrhizin, the part that may increase blood pressure, removed.

- **Boswellia:** Boswellia helps provide joint support and helps prevent arthritis. Some people suggest it as an herbal remedy for Crohn's disease, asthma, and colitis.

Choosing Dietary Supplements Wisely

More and more people are turning to nutritional supplements to either battle inflammatory issues they're at risk for or just give themselves a bit of a healthy boost. You can see evidence of the growing number of people looking for supplements on the store shelves: the number of companies producing supplements seems to grow every day.

But like pharmaceutical drugs, supplements present dangers of unsafe inter-actions or incorrect dosages. Despite all their healthy anti-inflammatory benefits, if you take too much of any supplement, you stand a good chance of doing more harm than good.

Trying to self-prescribe supplements and deciding on your dosage is dangerous. Always turn to a healthcare provider before starting any kind of supplement to make sure it's the right one for you and that it won't react with other medications, your diet, or anything else in your lifestyle.

In this section, we outline how an expert can help you decide which supplements to choose and how much to take. We also show you how to read labels correctly, so you know that what you're picking up is what you want.

Getting some professional guidance

Consult a naturopathic physician or other medical experts who are specially trained in nutrition and dietary and herbal supplements. Here are some things your Naturopath or other nutritional experts can help with:

- Which supplements are safe and effective: Drugs are tightly regulated by the Food and

Drug Administration (FDA) and must go through rigorous and expensive laboratory and clinical trials before they can be put on the market. However, because herbs and supplements do not require FDA approval, you rarely see much clinical research on their activity or benefits. An expert can tell you which supplements likely do what they're supposed to.

- A specific type of supplement: Maybe you read in a magazine that echinacea is good for colds. But did you know there are many species of echinacea and that not all of them work effectively as an immune system booster? A naturopathic physician has had at least four years' training in herbal medicine as part of his or her medical school education.

- Ingredients: You don't know what you're getting when you pick up supplements from someone other than a professional, and you can do more harm than good by taking a product over the counter. Fish oils, for example, are favorable for your heart and may help lower cholesterol, but taking a poor-quality fish oil may increase your cholesterol by causing further oxidation rather than preventing oxidation.

Your physician can guide you toward quality products. Sometimes quality means paying more for what you need, but the real question is this: Do you want to pay for your health now or later? If you penny-pinch on supplements, you may be setting yourself up to spend much more in hospital bills later.

- Possible interactions and side effects: Herbs and supplements, although generally safer than pharmaceutical drugs, do have potential side effects and can interact with other supplements and medications. An expert can tell you which supplements interact with medicines and can help you through any problems.

- Proper dosage: More isn't necessarily better. Ingesting too much of a specific vitamin or supplement can be dangerous. For example, some supplements may boast 500 percent of the recommended daily value of vitamin C. However, too much vitamin C can cause diarrhea and dehydration, and an abuse of some B vitamins can cause temporary nerve damage, including tingling in the hands and feet. Be sure to consider how much of each nutrient you're getting through your diet when determining the dosage of a supplement. Turn to your Naturopath or other medical professionals to find out how much to take.

- Individualized treatment: Your physician can help make sure you get the right combination for your genetics, biochemical individuality, and lifestyle. Just as your fingerprints are unique, so is the way your body works. Have a professional assess your case for an optimal treatment plan.

Not all states or Canadian provinces have licensure for naturopathic doctors, so some individuals use the title without the four-year medical education. Seek out a practitioner who got his or her degree from an accredited school and not an online program. Two websites that can help you find a licensed naturopathic doctor are www.naturopathic.org and www.cand.ca.

<u>**Understanding labels**</u>

After you consult with a physician (making sure you ask which retailers have the best quality supplements), pick up the bottle, look at the label, and ask these two key questions:

- Where do the nutrients come from? Like other food products, dietary supplements have a nutritional label with the ingredients listed. Some manufacturers put the source of the nutrient next to the ingredient.

  Recognize any of the names? You should be able to recognize and pronounce most, if not all, of the ingredients and sources.

- Does it have natural or artificial ingredients? Just as you don't want to eat artificial sugars or refined flours, you want your supplements to be natural with no artificial or chemical ingredients. Even when the ingredient is a derivative of the whole product, you're losing some value of the whole nutrient. For example, are there artificial colors or additives like sodium lauryl sulfate or propylene glycol?

These ingredients have no health benefits; they just make the product appear more appealing.

Considering quality standards

Not all supplements are created equal. Although pharmaceutical drugs have standardized formulas, supplements can vary in their composition. With whole-plant extracts, for example, the amount of the active constituent (effective ingredient) that the plant produces will vary; some companies created standardized extracts for this reason. There's controversy in the herbal medicine industry because sometimes the stated amount of the active compound is inaccurate, such as with hypericin in St. John's wort. Similarly, two bottles, both saying they contain ginger may have varying levels of actual ginger, supplemented themselves with chemicals or other additives in an effort to make the product — though not necessarily the ginger — last longer.

There are no strict standards (a few countries do have) on the quality of ingredients for nutritional supplements and herbs, so many products lack clinical effectiveness. The FDA (www.fda.gov) is trying to improve standards with its updated Dietary Supplements Health and Education Act (DSHEA) through improving good manufacturing practices (GMP). However, there's no substitute for expert advice.

When searching for the best quality supplements, take these first steps:

- Do your research. Go online and check reputable sources — the Better Business Bureau, the Food and Drug Administration, and the U.S. Department of Agriculture, for starters — to see what they may say about various herbs and supplements. Then check company websites — see what they say about their research and quality standards. Are they promoting the quality of the product or the fact that it's the cheapest on the market? Have their products been tested by an independent lab?

  If something sounds too good to be true, it probably is. If a supplement guarantees it will make you lose X number of pounds in 30 days, be wary. Every person's body responds to each supplement in its way; there's no real way to know for how long — or whether — a supplement will work for you. Be wary of anecdotal "testimonials" about amazing results or of anything that claims to be "totally safe."

- Look for the expiration date. It sounds like a simple step, but you'd be surprised by the number of people who don't realize supplements expire. Don't take expired supplements expecting to get the full nutritional value. Things that contain oils may go rancid beyond their effectiveness date, particularly if they've been exposed to heat and light.

- Check with the store. Avoid going to price clubs or pharmacies for nutritional supplements; you can generally find better-quality supplements in your physician's office or at a health food store. Your health-care provider should be recommending a specific brand. See what the health food stores on-duty nutritionist or other expert knows about a particular company or brand. If a product is of good quality, the staff will likely know about it. The quality of the product is generally reflected in the price.

Don't shop online for vitamins, herbs, or supplements. You don't know what you're getting, and a lot of scams are out there. Even though the label looks good, there's no guarantee the bottle will have anything useful in it.

FIGHTING INFLAMMATION WITH EXERCISE

Sticking to a regular high-intensity workout that is short — about 15 to 30 minutes — reduces your risks of obesity, and therefore, your risks of metabolic. Physical exercise is also associated with a decreased risk of cardiovascular and heart disease. Exercise promotes the release of feel-good endorphins, helps the immune system (when you do not overdo it), helps with weight loss and maintenance, and is a great stress reliever. Increased blood flow and sweating enhance detoxification, and exercise helps your body use sugars instead of storing them in the liver, which helps improve problems with insulin resistance.

Furthermore, building and maintaining lean muscle mass helps your metabolism to function optimally and helps reduce inflammation. Lean muscle mass, rather than fat, helps with inflammation because excess fat cells cause toxicity and inflammatory disruption in the signals of the endocrine system.

In this section, we introduce ways you can get the blood flowing and build a little muscle in the process.

Remember to stretch before and after every workout. Stretching has a way of fooling your muscles into thinking they are already or still working, enhancing the benefits of your exercise by up to 20 percent. Stretching also helps your muscles begin to contract more smoothly, alleviating some of the pain you may feel early on.

Starting simply with walking and swimming

Walking is the best place to start, mainly because it is something you likely do to some degree every day. Walking is an easy and excellent way to boost your heart rate, it is easier on your joints than running, and it is something you can do at any time. Walk around the house in inclement weather or go up and down the stairs a few times. Better yet, get a treadmill and walk for miles, even when it is raining.

The best way to make an exercise routine stick is to find a way to make it enjoyable. When you are walking, find a pleasant route with great things to see or one that makes you feel comfortable and relaxed. With other exercises, try playing some upbeat music or exercising with friends.

Integrate more walking into your routine by doing so gradually. Keep a pedometer handy and work weekly to boost the number of steps you take each day. If you are walking 2,000 steps now, for example, shoot for 2,500 next week. Keep that up for a week and then shoot for another 500-step boost.

Swimming is another excellent way to get your heart pumping. The waterworks soothe the joints rather than put extra stress on them, so swimming is therapeutic as well as aerobic. If you have access to a pool, try to incorporate 30 minutes of swimming into your routine three to four times a week.

When you get your body ready, you can step the workout up a notch, being sure to incorporate 30 minutes of exercise into your day at least three times a week.

Get it going well: Stimulating exercises

The following sections guide you through a few moves that are sure to get your heart going. Be sure to have an exercise mat and plenty of room to get the most out of your workout. Doing these exercises in a sequence is a great start to a good fitness routine, and altogether you will have about a 20-minute workout. Do not be afraid to do each exercise a little longer or find another to add to the routine if you want to stretch your workout to 30 minutes.

Squat thrusts

These squat thrusts are a great way to start your exercise routine and get your heart rate nice and high while working your entire body.

Stand with your feet about hip-width apart.

Squat to the floor, placing your hands directly in front of you and about shoulder-width apart.

With your weight on your arms, very quickly jump your feet behind you so that you are in a push-up position, then jump back and stand up.

Try to do 10 repetitions within a minute. Pause for 30 seconds and then do another set of 10. Pause for another 30 seconds and do a third set of 10.

If your inflammation is in your knees or hips, be sure to consult a physician before trying squat thrusts, and start with shorter, slower repetitions.

Mountain climbers

As with squat thrusts, mountain climbers raise your heart rate rather quickly.

Begin in a push-up position with your legs out straight.

Bring your right knee to your chest, resting your foot on the floor.

Quickly jump and switch legs, returning the right leg to a straight line and bringing the left knee up.

Continue alternating legs as quickly as you can for a full minute. Pause for 30 seconds and repeat for another minute. Take another 30-second break before doing a final minute of mountain climbers.

Be sure to consult a physician if your inflammation is in your legs because mountain climbers may exacerbate rather than relieve some of the pain.

Deep squat lunges

These lunges are great for raising your heart rate without the added pressure on your knees and hips. If you have inflammation in your legs, these lunges will aid in the healing process without risking re-injury.

Stand with your feet shoulder-width apart, arms at your sides.

Step your left foot out to the left, bending your left knee and extending your right leg in a side lunge.

As you lunge to the left, raise your right arm over your head and reach left. Bring your left arm across your hips and reach right. Be careful not to let your left knee extend past your toes.

Return to your starting position, with feet shoulder-width apart and arms at your sides.

Repeat step 2, this time lunging to the right and reaching your left arm up and over your head.

Return to your starting position.

Continue lunges for 5 minutes, alternating sides. Try to stretch a little farther with each lunge.

Invisible jump rope

This exercise raises your heart rate and lets you control how quickly it climbs based on how fast you jump.

Stand upright with your feet hip-width apart. Keeping elbows at your sides, pretend you are holding a jump rope.

Begin twirling the imaginary rope and jumping.

Continue for five minutes, varying speeds.

Be careful if you are having trouble with your knees because the bouncing can create a painful impact.

Slowing it down: Relaxing moves

Not quite ready for moving fast, or need something to help you cool down? Here are a few moves that keep your heart rate up without putting a strain on your joints.

Intermittent leg lifts

These leg lifts are a much less aerobic move than some exercises and therefore should not cause additional strain on any of your joints. It is an excellent starter move for people who suffer inflammation pain in the hips and or knees.

Lie on your back on your exercise mat, arms at your sides with hands flat.

Keeping your legs together, raise your feet 6 inches; hold them up for 10 seconds.

Pressing your hands to the floor for support, raise your feet another 6 inches and hold for 10 seconds.

Again, pressing your hands to the floor for support, raise your feet one more time, this time, so your legs and torso form a right angle; hold for 10 seconds.

Slowly begin lowering your feet, holding your feet 12 inches off the ground for 10 seconds and at 6 inches for 10 seconds.

When your feet are back on the floor, rest for 15 seconds and repeat. Perform this exercise four times.

After you get this move mastered, add some variation by holding a ball between your feet as you raise your legs. First, use a playground ball, and then up in size until eventually, you work with a stabilizer ball.

Stabilizing ab crunch

This ab crunch is a great exercise to help reduce some of that dangerous belly fat while at the same time increasing your heart rate. The stability ball provides support to your lower back.

Get out your stability ball and put it on the center of your exercise mat.

Stand in front of the ball with your feet at shoulder-width apart.

Lower yourself so that you are sitting on the ball.

Cross your arms over your chest or clasp your hands gently behind your head and lie back, letting your back curve slightly with the ball.

Slowly rise so that your shoulders come up off the ball.

Repeat. Do 10 crunches, slowing increasing by 5 crunches over time.

LEARN TO MANAGE PAIN WITH MINDSET TRAINING

Your gut health can influence your mental health through of the gut-brain pivot, yet this is not only a single direction association. Your mind, your thoughts, and your demeanor can likewise influence your physical and digestive health. If you need to adopt a holistic approach to take your fitness to the next level, you also need to think about what your thoughts can cause. Conventional allopathic medication tragically does not generally appear to focus on this part of the health condition, despite its essential, obvious significance.

Do not avoid this part on the off chance that you need to arrive at your full health potential. You do not have to adopt an altogether new, elusive practice to improve your mind-body association. Seemingly insignificant details like better dealing with your stress, setting aside effort for yourself, snickering, thinking positive thoughts, and sleeping deeply can make all the distinction in the world.

Stress and Digestive Health

Stress can and will keep you from progressing on your BYO diet, so do not make the mix-up of rejecting its significance. Regardless of whether you are doing everything right with your diet, not focusing on your mental health can be sufficient to propagate your digestive problems and point of confinement to your food resilience.

Stress can be acute (present moment) or chronic (long term). It very well may be passionate or physical. A wide range of stress can be problematic for your digestive health. Familiar sources of stress incorporate cutoff times, exhausting, money related concerns, interpersonal clashes, and not getting enough sleep or downtime. If you have a sort A personality and are always searching for something to do, you are particularly prone to stress. Indeed, even positive forms of stress can trigger a stress response in your body. Voyaging, starting another relationship, getting hitched, starting a family, or taking up a new position can be similarly stressful for your body.

Physical forms of stress can likewise have negative ramifications for your health. Over the top exercise (particularly continuance exercise), just as pain, infection, gastrointestinal problems, or food sensitivities would all be able to compromise your progress. Energizers like caffeine can likewise put additional stress on your body.

WHY IS STRESS SO PROBLEMATIC?

Your body has a switch that allows it to work in two unique modes: parasympathetic or thoughtful. Your parasympathetic mode ought to be your default mode. That is the rest and digest mode that allows your body to do fix and upkeep work. This mode is additionally liable for setting the conditions for healthy digestion. It is just when your parasympathetic mode is enacted that you can produce stomach acid, digestive enzymes, and bile to encourage assimilation and assist you with bettering the retention of the nutrients from your food.

Numerous people have disabled digestion because stress turns their body switch to thoughtful mode. In this battle or flight mode, in addition to the fact that metabolism is inhibited, stress hormones like cortisol and adrenaline are emitted in enormous sums. This response is totally typical and even fundamental in instances of acute stress to set you up to face potential threats. The problem is that our sensory system was manufactured mostly to confront transient stressors like chasing for food or fleeing from predators. The stress response started by the thoughtful sensory system makes you prepared to face the situation by making you progressively alert so you can react by either battling or fleeing. The type of stress we tend to experience today is more chronic nature, preventing our bodies from returning to their default parasympathetic mode that facilitates proper digestion and healing. The elevated cortisol levels associated with the activation of your sympathetic mode can also:

- Disrupt your sleep;

- Fatigue your adrenal glands;

- Contribute to blood-sugar regulation problems;

- Promote weight gain around your waist;

- Alter your gut flora;

- Downregulate your immune system;

- Promote inflammation;

- Inhibit cleansing waves (essential to preventing overgrowth of microorganisms in your small intestines);

- Increase intestinal permeability (causing leaky gut and leading to many digestive and systemic symptoms, as well as multiple food sensitivities).

Everyone deals with stress in his or her daily life. You cannot avoid stress, but what you can change is how you react to and cope with it. You cannot try to manage your stress only once a month, though. You need to cultivate stress management and relaxation on a daily basis, just like a garden that needs to be tended every day. If you do not keep the weeds under control, your flowers will not bloom.

Remember that your mind and body are intimately connected. Do not ignore your mental health, or your physical health may plateau and even relapse instead of reaching its full potential. Cultivating a positive attitude is not always easy when you suffer from chronic GI issues, but it is important to focus on the positive. While it may be challenging to feel good about bloating, diarrhea, and constipation, focus on the positive changes you are making and feel empowered by what you have already learned about digestive health. You now better understand what is at the root of your symptoms, and you know how to use a REAL-food-based elimination diet to say goodbye to your symptoms and recover your digestive health. You are taking charge of your health, and things can and will get better soon. It will take some work, but you are closer to optimal digestive health than you ever were.

You have the opportunity to overcome your digestive problems, or at least improve them significantly if you only give yourself a chance. Focus on the relationships and other positive elements in your life, however small they may seem. It does not have to be something big: a pet that is always there for you, a sunny day, or the fresh smell of rain. If you cannot think of anything positive, make something positive happen. Buy yourself flowers, treat yourself to a massage, or indulge in some quiet meditation.

Techniques to Tend Your Inner Garden

What else can you do to manage your stress, besides quitting your job and spending the rest of your life on a desert island? You can implement small strategies as part of your daily routine to cultivate a healthy mind and put your body in rest-and-digest mode. Maintaining a positive attitude alone is already a significant improvement, but you can also include a few simple, quick relaxation techniques in your daily routine.

All you need is five to 10 minutes once or twice a day (and if you can dedicate more time, even better). Every minute you take to nurture your mind garden will help to keep out the weeds and allow your flowers to bloom. The following techniques only take a few minutes and can offer huge benefits to your mental and bodily health:

- Belly breathing;

- Finding a secret "happy place";

- Spending time with Mother Nature;

- Body scanning;

- Making a gratitude list;

- Finding a hobby;

- Laughing;

- Smiling.

PRACTICE BELLY BREATHING

Lie down on your bed, on your couch, or outside on the grass. You can also sit if you prefer. Close your eyes, place your hands on your lower abdomen, and try to breathe only with your belly by making it inflate and deflate like a balloon as you breathe in and out. Your chest shouldn't move too much. It might feel a bit awkward at first, but you'll get used to it. While breathing in, count from one to seven, in your head or aloud. Hold your breath for one count then count down from eight to zero while breathing out, trying to push all the air out of your lungs.

Breathe as slowly and as deeply as you can. If you prefer, you can omit the counting and repeat a mantra word or phrase with each respiration. Or simply imagine your breath as a light that fills your body each time you inspire. Try to do belly-breathing exercises for at least five minutes, but 15 to 20 minutes is ideal for getting a maximal reinvigorating effect.

FIND A SECRET "HAPPY PLACE"

You can do this exercise anywhere. Make yourself comfortable, lying down, or sitting as you prefer. Close your eyes and think of a place or moment in your life that made you happy. Imagine the setting in your head, what it looked like, how it felt, what you heard, what you smelled, the people who were with you. It could be a vacation place, a nature spot, or the site of a special celebration.

Try to relive the moment you chose, as if you're watching a favorite movie. You can even adjust your memory to make it more exciting or enjoyable—or create one from scratch! Just make sure you imagine every detail to make it as real as possible. Do this for as long or as short as you like. Anytime you feel stressed, close your eyes for a minute or two and conjure this happy place to help you feel more relaxed and address your stress.

SPEND TIME WITH MOTHER NATURE

Nature can have a powerful, calming effect. Unfortunately, too many people spend most of their lives inside their homes, classrooms, offices, and cars. All you need to experience the invigorating power of nature is a little piece of grass, ideally with a few trees. It could be in your backyard, a city park, or even on a beach. Lie down or sit in the grass and enjoy the nature around you. Try not to think too much, letting your thoughts come and go without focusing on any single one. Instead, pay attention to the sensations you experience. Like the wind, you are feeling the sun's warmth on your skin, the smells, and the sounds around you. Feel your body being supported by the stable ground underneath you.

Try to keep some parts of your skin in direct contact with the grass or sand. Earthing, or the practice of being directly in connection with the ground, has been shown in various studies to decrease stress, regulate cortisol levels, lower inflammation, and promote better sleep. You can also get the same grounding benefits by taking a walk barefoot or swimming in a lake or the ocean. Going outside to relax will also give you the bonus of getting some vitamin D. It may be a bit more challenging to practice earthing during winter in some areas. However, you can still enjoy the fresh air and Mother Nature's calming effect by taking a walk or sitting in a quiet park.

PRACTICE BODY SCANNING

Lie down or sit somewhere comfortably. Close your eyes and scan your body, body part by body part. One by one, slowly contract each muscle group of your body starting from your face, neck, shoulders, upper arms, lower arms, hands, and fingers, without moving. Move to your chest, back, and abdomen before attending to your glutes, thighs, calves, feet, and toes. Doing the cycle once is enough to feel more relaxed, but you can repeat it as often as you'd like to deepen the relaxation.

MAKE A GRATITUDE LIST

Experiencing gratitude is a great way to feel calm and relaxed. Feeling appreciative results in the release of the hormone oxytocin, which activates your parasympathetic nervous system and switches your body into its rest-and-digest mode. You can enable gratitude by creating a "gratitude list" of everything you're thankful for: the meaningful relationships in your life, your ability to take charge of your health by changing the way you eat, and even the restful sleep you had the night before. You can be grateful for things you've done, things that have happened to you, or things you've received. Keep this list on your fridge or bedside table, or somewhere else you can see it, and read it as often as you need. Add more items as you think of them. Whenever you feel stressed, focus on one of the things on your list for a few minutes.

Instead of a list, you can also write all the things for which you're thankful on separate pieces of paper and put them in a jar. Whenever you feel down, open the jar and pick one to cheer you up. Hold on to the gratitude as long as you can to help you feel calmer and more centered.

LAUGH!

Laughing is a serious matter. It oxygenates your body, stimulates circulation, and encourages the release of feel-good hormones (endorphins) that can calm you down and make you feel better quickly. Laughter can even boost your immune system. Most people understand the importance of not taking life too seriously, and that laughing is functional, but not many make it a regular exercise.

Try simply laughing for three to five minutes straight. You don't have to be laughing at anything; faking it counts. Even if you feel ridiculous during this exercise, do it at least once to experience the powerful effect of laughter. Alternate between vowel sounds and adjust the loudness and quality of your laughter as you like. It can be hard to do at first, but you'll feel amazingly relaxed afterward—and you'll likely want to do it again soon.

Whenever you face a stressful situation, try to respond by — yep — laughing. Laughing can help you detach yourself from the negative emotions associated with the situation. Laugh out the stress!

SMILE

Some researchers believe that emotions are activated by facial expressions rather than the other way around. The simple act of smiling, even a forced smile, can send a message to your body and mind that triggers the release of important calming and relaxing hormones. If you don't feel like laughing, or you're in an environment where laughing wouldn't be appropriate, just smile. Do this in your car, on your way to work, while working on your computer, during a meeting or exam, or while talking to friends.

FIND A HOBBY

Most people are too busy or believe they are too busy to take the time for hobbies they once enjoyed. Hobbies are a fantastic way to adjust your mind frame and forget about the stresses in your life. If you find you're not as interested in collecting stamps or stickers as you did when you were 11, try taking up a new pastime. It could be dancing, listening to music or playing an instrument, scrapbooking, drawing, photography, jewelry making, woodworking, knitting, model building, studying a foreign language, rock climbing, gardening, writing, or reading (ideally not health-or nutrition-related!). Whatever you choose, make sure it's something that helps you feel more relaxed and take your mind off your worries.

DO WHAT MAKES YOU FEEL GOOD

Experiment with these relaxation methods to see which ones you prefer. Write down a list of your favorite techniques and put it on your fridge to remind you of all the great tools you've developed to help combat stress. You can even try combining the techniques. Try to do some belly breathing while smiling or thinking of a particular place that makes you feel calm and relaxed. Or take a nature walk while recalling items from your gratitude list. There are no rules, except no stressing about any of it! You deserve to spend a bit of time every day doing what makes you feel good and happy.

ADDRESS STRESSFUL SITUATIONS HEAD-ON

It's essential to take time on a regular basis to practice the techniques above, just like you need to tend your garden frequently to prevent weeds from suffocating your flowers. But what should you do when confronted with an immediately stressful situation? Whenever a stressful situation arises, remember to stay calm. That might be easier said than done, but the more you practice, the better at it you will become. With any problem, there are always three things you can do to resolve it:

- Change the situation,

- Adapt yourself to the situation, or

- Leave the situation.

How would this work in practice? Let's say that work is a significant source of stress in your life. What can you do? You can either try changing the situation by talking to your supervisor about making deadlines more reasonable or trying to find ways to make your workload easier to manage. If you can't change the situation directly, you can adapt yourself to it by changing your attitude toward your work. Instead of feeling like your job is a chore or torture, try looking at it as a challenge. Try to adopt a positive attitude by recognizing how your job helps you get the money you need to afford beautiful things and better appreciate the time you spend outside the office. If neither of these strategies works, the job is making your life miserable and interfering with your quality of life and your health, try to find another job that would be a better fit for you. You have options. Don't be a victim and take control of your life.

GET ENOUGH QUALITY SLEEP

Many studies emphasize the importance of sleep for optimal health. Lack of sleep can compromise your learning and memory, mood, weight, cardiovascular health, and immune system, and can even trigger cravings. A single night of poor sleep can induce insulin resistance in healthy people, which constitutes a risk factor and a first step toward developing type 2 diabetes and heart disease.

Not getting enough sleep can also be perceived as a stress by your body and result in the same harmful consequences for your digestive health caused by any other type of anxiety. Insomnia can also be a sign of adrenal fatigue, and one can worsen the other in a vicious cycle. You need good sleep to allow your body and digestive system to heal and function optimally, so you have to make sleep a priority.

You need between eight and nine hours of sleep every night, so make sure you go to bed at the right time, ideally before 9:30-10 PM. If you have trouble falling asleep, make sure you turn off the lights or keep them to a minimum one or two hours before bedtime. Turn off the television and stay away from the computer. Too much light interferes with the release of hormones like melatonin that makes you naturally sleepy within a few hours after the sunset. To avoid interfering with these hormones, use the last hour or two before your bedtime to read by a small table lamp, take a bath or shower, or just relax to help your body get ready for a good night's sleep.

Light is what synchronizes your body's natural rhythm. Humans are meant to go to sleep within a few hours after the sun goes down and wake up when the sun rises (varying according to the time of the year). Artificial light disrupts this normal cycle by causing insomnia or preventing you from getting restorative sleep. Try to get some natural sunshine during the day to help your body know it's daytime, and make your room as dark as you can at night, so your body gets the message that it is nighttime. Cover up your windows as best you can and remove any night lights, alarm clocks, or other light sources in your room since they can interfere with sleep hormones.

At the point when we talk about inflammation, incidentally, we're talking about systemic inflammation - cellular inflammation. It's not equivalent to curving your lower leg and afterward seeing the restricted swelling that results.

The inflammation we're talking about here is undeniably progressively slippery. It resembles a chronic irritant to our bodies and psyches, like a fire discreetly seething inside.

It's of particular significance to address inflammation of the gut. The gut is unpredictably attached to the brain and brain work, as bleeding-edge logical research keeps on illustrating. A "bad gut rises to a bad brain." Consider the potential for even more precisely and effectively treating (or anticipating) conditions like melancholy, tension, range disorders, Alzheimer's, etc. The gut must not be overlooked.

So, what causes inflammation?

Here are the absolute most common factors related to inflammation:

1. Diet - Eating "inflammatory" foods, particularly grains like wheat, grain, and rye that contain gluten and present inflammatory proteins called prolamins. These chronically disturb the gut and contribute to gut penetrability or "leaky gut." When the gut is too permeable, huge molecules that were never planned to pass through the intestinal barrier are allowed to do as such. That triggers an over-dynamic immune response as the immune system goes on the attack. One

of the results of this uplifted immune response is inflammation.

2. Sugar - Whether it's the white fine, precious stone stuff right off the spoon, or out of a bundle, or it's foods and drinks that break down to sugar quickly in our bloodstream (like juice, pop, desserts and dull carbs like bread, pasta, grain, saltines, pizza, baked goods, and cakes), sugar spikes create a negative response no matter how you look at it. Blood sugar dysregulation from chronic sugar spikes and insulin obstruction are immediate supporters of inflammation. Artificial sugars are not an answer! These are highly toxic and contribute to inflammation too.

3. "Bad" Fats - Another dietary guilty party are the trans fats. Hydrogenated and partially hydrogenated fats, business vegetable oils, the fat from tainted animal sources, abundance omega-6 fats and oils, etc. These contribute to an inflammatory condition. Stick with unadulterated coconut oil, good grass-

bolstered spread, natural additional virgin olive oil. Use healthy fats from grass-sustained and unfenced creature sources, wild fish, healthy fat foods like avocado, an equalization of omega-3 to omega-6 fats, etc. The "bad" fats are what we usually get with lousy nourishment, cheap food, restaurant food, seared foods, etc. In any event, when we start with "healthy" food, when we cook it with bad fats, the results are toxic and inflammatory.

4. Leaky Gut and Autoimmune Conditions - I know I just mentioned it. However, it needs its clear spot on this list. It's an endless loop: leaky gut leads to inflammation, which in turn leads to the leaky gut, and that leads to even more inflammation. You get the point. This loop is an immune response. The immune system is merely carrying out its responsibility of attacking things that shouldn't be there, as too-enormous molecules passing through the intestinal barrier. At the point when this cycle proceeds, the stage is splendidly set for an autoimmune condition. As the immune

response proceeds on its attack "against" the body. The insightful approach to remedying this isn't to stifle the general immune response, yet to (1) expel the triggers, accordingly 'calming' the immune response, and (2) recuperate the gut.

5. Stress - Whether it's mental, enthusiastic, or physical, chronic stress assumes an immediate job in cellular inflammation. Our bodies are flawlessly fit for short sessions of stress - it's known as the "battle or flight response." In any case, when we're chronically presented to stress, systems break down. Reasons can be due to continuous money-related issues, relationship challenges, vocation disappointment, chronic sleep deprivation, injury, over-working, over-preparing (for example, for a long-distance race), drugs, toxic foods. There's no lack of stressors! Stress creates a remarkable course of neuro-hormonal occasions in the brain and body that simply can't be overlooked.

6. Toxicity - We are immersed with toxicity. Some of it, our body can adjust to. Some of it, we can't. Toxicity triggers a particular chemical/hormonal response in the brain and sets off a chain of occasions all through the whole body. Inflammation is one of them. Take a gander at the list about in the "stress" class - those are altogether sources of toxicity. To that list, we can include environmental toxicity also. Think about sources of toxicity from air, water, personal consideration products, family unit, nursery, and grass care products, makeup, overwhelming metals, antibodies, and so on. It very well may be overwhelming to think about how toxic our world has become. It's the reason I accept that a conventional cellular detoxification protocol is so important.

7. Chronic Sleep Deprivation - Hopefully, you can see the association here. Deprivation (or inadequacy) anyplace along with the range of 'things our body needs' can lead to a toxic, inflamed circumstance. Be that as it may, even

one night of sleep deprivation (we're talking 4 - 5 hours of sleep here) has been shown to raise the markers of inflammation essentially!

8. Chronic Alcohol Consumption - Alcohol contributes to leaky gut, just as bacterial and contagious/yeast abundance in the intestines. It's a highly thought portion of sugar, also setting off the body's insulin response.

9. Medication Use - Many remedy and over-the-counter medications legitimately contribute to inflammation themselves. One of these is NSAIDS (non-steroidal anti-inflammatory medications, similar to headache medicine, ibuprofen, Celebrex, and so forth). Research undeniably demonstrates that even 3 days of assuming over-the-counter control medications like ibuprofen can cause inflammation and a leaky gut. Another family tranquilizes straightforwardly connected to gut inflammation is antibiotics. Antibiotics don't just attack the proposed target bacteria - they unleash destruction on all bacteria, including the "healthy" bacteria all through

our intestinal systems that are so basic to our general wellbeing and immune capacity.

10. Dietary Deficiencies - As I referred to before, lack implies we're not getting what our cells require to accomplish and keep up a condition of homeostatic cell work. This condition can lead to inflammation as a result of the absence of key 'fixings' required for proper digestion.

11. Low Hydrochloric Acid in the Stomach - Most people feel that indigestion and acid reflux are the results of having a lot of acid in the stomach. With this considered, more often than not, it's the exact inverse, particularly as we get more seasoned. At the point when we need more HCL to break down our food properly, we can encounter the consuming sensation as particles of food that are not correctly separated remain in the upper digestive tract for longer than they should. The body is stating, "Hello, this food is too enormous for me to pass along to the small intestines!" Or on the other hand, if those food particles that are too enormous do get passed

on to the small intestine, they cause the breakdown of the intestinal coating, leading to leaky gut, which causes chronic inflammation.

Things being what they are, those acid pump inhibiting drugs you see on TV? They wind up, causing the food to be pushed out of the stomach before it's processed properly. This way, you quit feeling the burn. However, now you've made way for a lot of more concerning issues with gut penetrability, leaky gut, inflammation, and making way for an autoimmune condition after some time.

12. Hormonal Imbalance - This is a major one! We're not simply talking about reproductive hormones, or "women's" hormones, which numerous people still expect when you mention "hormonal"! Hormones are the chemical couriers for every one of the systems of our bodies, and they assume a primary job in each capacity. One case of the hormonal-inflammation association is with the stress hormone, cortisol.

At the point when our adrenal system is fatigued from chronic stress or toxicity, we can burn through such an extensive amount, our stress hormone supply that cortisol gets exhausted. Sadly, cortisol is something that our body uses to control the inflammatory process, typically!

On the other side, when there is inflammation, the hormonal receptors on the cell film end up not being so 'open' to the hormonal message endeavoring to be delivered. That is the result of hormonal dysregulation - the message can't get to its proposed goal, or the message gets slanted. A hormone medication or cream doesn't illuminate this difficulty.

13. Infections - Bacterial, viral, contagious, or parasitic. These chronic, regularly undetected and untreated, infections cause inflammation as the immune system is tirelessly on the attack, attempting to monitor the infection. Perhaps the easiest thing we can do to counterbalance potential infection, particularly in the gut, is to recharge the gut

with healthy, immune enabling bacteria as high-quality probiotics.

14. Extreme Brain Trauma - Remember the underlying association between the gut and the brain? Here, it happens backward. When there is a brain injury, it has been shown that it causes leaky gut in as meager as six hours or less! As we know by now, this leads to chronic inflammation after some time if not adequately tended to.

While this list can appear to be overwhelming and difficult to survive, it's most certainly not. We can change to an increasingly "anti-inflammatory" lifestyle without hardly lifting a finger.

Remember, however, the "anti-inflammatory" approach will just get you up until this point. You've additionally got the chance to recuperate and fix the gut. Generally, the inflammatory cycle can proceed indeed, even in response to "healthy" choices in diet, for instance.

Please don't fuss! It's not tied in with being great. It's tied in with settling on better choices, more regularly.

Stick to "genuine" food versus manufactured factory foods and low-quality nourishment, remain hydrated, move your body, add something like yoga to sustain your general health, have an outlet for stress, get enough sleep, be thankful, evacuate the same number of sources of toxicity as you can... everything is great!

Each healthy decision signifies to make a positive contrast, and you'll always be unable to remove a healthy choice that you made! Simply focus and connect some of them (the more, the better) every day, every week, for the long run. That's how health is created and maintained.

FIGHTING INFLAMMATION WITH MEDITATION AND YOGA

Everybody experiences a little stress, and when you're confronting health issues or rolling out huge improvements, that stress level can slowly inch upward until you feel tense, anxious, and out and out awkward. Stress is a cause of inflammation; when a lot of it occurs for a quite a long time, your body's characteristic anti-inflammatory hormone, cortisol, escapes balance.

For ages, people have utilized meditation and yoga to help the body typically relieve stress and get focused and loose.

Centering yourself through meditation

Avoiding all stress is incomprehensible; however, knowing how to manage stress helps make the bunch appear to be a lot smaller. For quite a long time, relaxation specialists have gone to centering, a form of meditation that includes deep breathing, slowing down your heart rate, and loosening up your muscles. Meditation can help lower blood pressure and relieve sleep deprivation and anxiety by reducing adrenaline levels and expanding the measure of serotonin released into the body. Serotonin, the "upbeat hormone," assumes a key job in deciding the state of mind and anxiety levels — the more serotonin, the better the temperament and the lower the anxiety.

In addition to the fact that meditation allows you to take a break from your day to calm your mind and body, research likewise shows that meditation counteracts pre-experienced maturing of the brain — the impacts of growing on things like memory, intellectual capacity, and responses.

Setting up and breathing

The initial phase in getting ready for an ideal meditation is to guarantee you have a spotless, calm space. Meditation is a way of cleaning up your mind, so make sure the area around you isn't loaded up with a mess either.

Lay your exercise tangle out flat. Light a scented candle or some incense, or utilize a couple of drops of essential oil in a diffuser to assist turn with bringing down the stress, and your inflammation along with it. Lavender helps with sleep and relaxation, and sandalwood can help with meditation.

Sit with your back straight and your feet flat on the floor. Close your eyes and take three deep, slow breaths. Focus your mind on your feet; imagine them slowly sending roots into the ground. As you breathe out, imagine yourself sending all your negative energy down through the roots into the earth. With each breath, imagine bringing positive energy up from the ground into your body. Picture the positive energy coming to you as white light, cresting on your crown.

Proceed with this breathing exercise until you feel your stress levels lowering.

Chakra

The chakra meditation is a breathing exercise where
you focus on different chakras, or part of your body,
with each purifying breath. The chakra — the Hindu
word for "wheel" or "turning" — is the idea of force
centers, turning receptors of energy permeating the
layers of the body.

Various systems have a differing number of chakras,
yet the most mainstream in the Western world is the
system of seven chakras (you start with the first):

- Base of the spine;

- Sexual organs;

- Stomach;

- Heart;

- Throat.

Head

While doing a chakra meditation, begin by laying
your yoga tangle out flat and lighting a scented
candle or some incense. Lavender helps with sleep

and relaxation, and sandalwood can help with meditation. Sit or rest with your back straight and your feet flat on the floor. Close your eyes and take three deep, slow breaths.

After you're loose, imagine a beautiful ball of energy pushing up through the earth and to your spine (the first chakra). The shade of the light is up to you, yet it ought to be a shading that you feel speaks to your energy.

As you breathe, imagine the ball of energy drifting over each of your chakras, purifying the area of negative energy, and boosting it with positive energy and relaxation. With each stop, the ball drives the antagonism up toward the sky.

At the point when you arrive at the seventh chakra, the head, let go of your ball of light and feel positive energy — a feel-decent factor — pushing up through you, again through the chakra process. Positive energy originates from focusing on positive things and pushing negative musings from your mind.

Going with the flow: Enjoying yoga

Yoga is a form of exercise that consolidates physical capacity with mind relaxation. Enjoying yoga all the time can make you feel physically better as well as sincerely more grounded, too.

Most Westernized yoga focuses on the physical stances of yoga or the asanas. These asanas stretch your muscles and help release the development of lactic acids, which cause fatigue, pain, and pressure. Perhaps the most significant advantage of yoga is its impact on the heart: By lowering blood weight and slowing the heart rate, yoga can help counteract different kinds of heart disease and heart attacks. It additionally helps lighten back pain and symptoms of asthma.

You can discover an assortment of yoga stances and levels of multifaceted nature, so feel free to experiment until you find out moves that work best for you. Here are the two types of stances we present in this section:

- Seated yoga presents: Seated stances are good for grounding and centering, and they're suitable for the beginning because they "open" the muscles for more extensive movement later; these stances incorporate the Butterfly, Lotus, and One Leg Forward Bend.

- Standing yoga presents: Standing postures are lively and great for assembling quality and parity; they incorporate Downward Dog, Tree, and Eagle.

Butterfly

Sit on your mat with your back straight. Unite your feet and bend your knees, lifting your knees slightly off the ground. Hold your feet or lower legs.

Lotus

The Lotus is probably one of the more known yoga positions. Sit leg over leg on your mat with your back straight. Slowly place your left foot onto your right thigh, and afterward place your right foot onto your left thigh. Rest your hands on your knees.

One Leg Forward Bend

Sit with your knees to your chest. Slowly stretch one leg out straight, while bending the other leg, allowing the knee to tumble off to the side and with your foot reaching your internal thigh. Hold for 20 seconds and afterward switch.

Descending Dog

Start on your hands and knees. Make sure your shoulders are over your wrists, and your knees are hip separation apart. Lift your hips and straighten your arms and legs, broadening your body into a great topsy turvy V shape. Note: Straighten your legs just to the extent is agreeable to you.

Tree

While standing, shift all your weight to one foot. At that point, lift the other foot and place it on your standing leg, on your internal thigh, or as high as you're able to put it. Never mind if it's only on your calf. Lift your arms straight over your head.

<u>**Eagle**</u>

Start in a standing position and shift all your weight to one foot. Bend your knee slightly and lift your other leg, folding it around and around your other leg. Snare the highest point of your foot around your calf. Enclose your arms by a wound position before you.